Lifting the Spirits

ALSO BY PENELOPE ODY

And available from Souvenir Press

Joint Pains

Sage

NATURE'S REMEDIES

Lifting the Spirits

Nature's Remedies for Stress and Relaxation

Penelope Ody, MNIMH

SOUVENIR PRESS

First published 2003 by
Souvenir Press Ltd,
43 Great Russell Street,
London WC1B 3PD

ISBN 0 285 63649 9

Typeset by Photoprint, Torquay, Devon
Printed and bound in Great Britain by Creative Print and Design Group (Wales), Ebbw Vale

Note to readers

The aim of this book is to provide information on the uses of herbs suitable for treating anxiety, stress and relaxation. Although every care has been taken to ensure that the advice is accurate and practical, it is not intended to be a guide to self-diagnosis and self-treatment. A number of the traditional herbs mentioned are now banned substances and their inclusion in this book is not intended as an endorsement for their use.

Where health is concerned – and in particular a serious problem of any kind – it must be stressed that there is no substitute for seeking advice from a qualified medical or herbal practitioner. All persistent symptoms, of whatever nature, may have underlying causes that need, and should not be treated without, professional elucidation and evaluation.

It is therefore very important, if you are considering trying herbal remedies for stress-related disorders, to consult your practitioner first, and if you are already taking any prescribed medication, to continue with this treatment.

The Publisher makes no representation, express or implied, with regard to he accuracy of the information contained in this book, and legal responsibility or liability cannot be accepted by the Author or Publisher for any errors or omissions that may be made or for any loss, damage, injury or problems suffered in any way arising from following the advice offered in these pages.

NOTE TO READERS

NB: Common names of herbs are used throughout the book. Botanical names are given for each main herbal entry in Chapters 2 and 4 where plants are listed in order of botanical name. A full cross-index of botanical names and common names is included as an Appendix.

Contents

Preface

It has become fashionable in recent years to blame many of our ills on 'stress'. We work long hours, juggling the demands of home, family and employer – not always successfully. At the same time our television screens deliver seemingly endless news of strife, famine or man's inhumanities. Small wonder that so many feel anxious, tense and less than optimistic about the future.

Stress can be defined in physiological terms as an inappropriate 'adrenaline rush'; it may be linked with food intolerance, or regarded as the result of unhappiness or mental anguish. 'Stress' may be dismissed as purely imaginary by some physicians or welcomed as a catch-all explanation for illness by others.

However we choose to regard 'stress', it is seen by many as the twenty-first-century's *bête noire,* closely associated with nervous problems: anxiety, panic attacks, emotional upsets, exhaustion, tension headaches, or depression. These problems certainly afflicted earlier generations – but often without that catch-all label of being 'stress-related'. As such we have a wealth of traditional herbal remedies used for centuries to combat the ills that we now blame on 'stress'.

Many of these remedies were used as preventatives: chewing coca or guarana to allay hunger and fatigue; drinking kava or smoking tobacco to encourage a relaxed ambience to ease social tensions. Mis-use of these remedies means that many are also now condemned as potentially bad for our health, like tobacco or even St John's wort, or banned entirely – as kava has recently been. Fortunately we still have many herbs to choose from to ease our tensions.

This book looks at the role herbs have played over the centuries in combating anxiety and depression; it reviews those that can be most effective and suggests suitable treatments for some of the many 'stress-related' ailments that the twenty-first-century is heir to. I hope you find it useful.

Penelope Ody
February 2003

CHAPTER 1

Soothing life's stresses

> He who is of a calm and happy nature will hardly feel the pressure of age, but to him who is of an opposite disposition, youth and age are equally a burden.
>
> Plato, *c.* 428–348BC

Stress is one of the twenty-first-century's greatest bugbears: blamed for an array of physical illnesses, domestic discord, workplace problems and generally dysfunctional lifestyles.

Yet, stress is a normal and necessary part of our lives: it provides a stimulus for activity and invention. Our bodies are equipped to deal with stress: our hormonal system springs into action to produce extra supplies of the hormone adrenaline to give us the energy for 'flight or fight' in difficult situations. Stress is part of being alive – without it we cease to function. But that so-called 'adrenaline rush' not only gears the body for action, it also gives us a euphoric 'high' which is potentially addictive and can be damaging in the long term.

That 'flight or fight' response is fine if we can do either of these actions, but if we don't the body remains over-active, in a constant state of alertness and that adds to feelings of frustration and a sense of being overloaded. This is what is commonly labelled as 'stress' but is more accurately the 'negative stress response'. If this response gets out of hand it can also be extremely damaging for health and increases the risk of a wide range of life-threatening diseases.

There are numerous widely accepted physical symptoms of stress while some health specialists argue that an inability to cope with stress can manifest in almost any sort of illness: a sudden cold as an excuse to take a day off work; frozen shoulder from an inability to 'fight' and punch that irritating work colleague; an unsightly skin disease sending out a protective 'keep away' message; or life-threatening diseases such as cancer and heart failure.

Common physical symptoms of an inability to cope with stress can involve:

- dry mouth
- palpitations (an awareness of one's heartbeat)
- constant tiredness
- difficulties with sleep and concentration
- an inability to relax and unwind
- recurring headaches
- muscular aches and pains
- diarrhoea or stomach upsets
- easy tears, or
- a tendency to feel low, in severe cases leading to depressive illness.

Some people seem to thrive on stress – happily juggling a dozen tasks with boundless energy. Others simply wilt. The trick is to find the stress level that best suits your particular temperament and energy and stay with it. More stress and you'll risk ill health; less and you may feel empty, bored and unfulfilled.

Social scientists have rated the various stresses to which we may all be exposed at various times (Table 1) and although many of the more mundane happenings have a low value, their repetition and cumulative effect can be dramatic. Regular demands from superiors (23 points), for example, will soon push up the stress quota. According to Dr Thomas Holmes, who devised one of the most widely used stress scales, if the total stress burden last year was more than 300, there is an 80 per cent chance of illness during

Table 1: The stress of life events (Holmes, 1967)

Event	Value
1. Death of a spouse	100
2. Getting divorced	73
3. Marriage separation	65
4. Going to prison	63
5. Death of a close family member	63
6. Major personal injury or illness	53
7. Marriage	50
8. Getting fired	47
9. Marital reconciliation	45
10. Retirement	45
11. Major change in health or behaviour of a family member	44
12. Pregnancy	40
13. Sexual difficulties	39
14. Gaining new family member (by birth, relatives arriving etc)	39
15. Major business readjustment	39
16. Major changes in finances (for better or worse)	38
17. Death of a close friend	37
18. Changing to a different type of work	36
19. A major change in the pattern of arguments with your partner (for better or worse)	35
20. Taking out a mortgage	31
21. Foreclosure on a mortgage or loan	30
22. A major change in responsibility at work	29
23. Child leaving home	29
24. Trouble with in-laws	29
25. Outstanding personal achievement	28
26. Partner starting or stopping work outside the home	26
27. Starting or completing formal schooling	26
28. Major change in living conditions	25
29. Significant change in personal habits, such as dress	24
30. Problems with employers	23
31. Major changes in working hours or conditions	20
32. Changing to a new school	20
33. Change in recreation habits	19
34. Major change in social activities	18
35. Taking out a loan	17
36. A change in sleeping habits	16
37. Major change in eating habits	15
38. Going on holiday	13
39. Christmas	12

the current year. With a level of 150–299 the risk is about 50 per cent. Under 150, and only around one in three will become ill. Keeping stress events to the minimum is clearly good for your health.

Western Society in the twenty-first century provides yet more opportunities for stress overload. For many the expression 'time poor, cash rich' is a very apt description of their lifestyles. There is never time to stand and stare, to relax and do nothing – life is a helter-skelter dash from work to play and back again. The 'escalator' analogy is common – we're on the moving stairway going in a predetermined direction and the act of changing course requires positive action. We're working longer, more fragmented hours, without the support that the extended family once provided. Modern technology may have given us automatic washing machines, ready-meals and electronic shopping on the Internet – but it has yet to do the ironing, stack the groceries in the larder, or solve our emotional problems.

The time rush simply increases feelings of inadequacy and tension: we live in a society which implies we 'can have it all' – the brilliant career, the happy family life, the socialising and leisure activities. And if work and household chores were not enough there is 'self-fulfilment'. Today it is simply not politically correct to curl up with a pulp novel and a stiff drink at the end of a hard day – the pressure is on to spend time expanding our horizons: learning a new language at evening classes, studying Tibetan chanting, taking an Open University degree or attempting to fathom the mysteries of *Feng Shui* and re-energise our homes.

Modern Western society is also characterised by a deep chasm separating our physical and spiritual dimensions. The divide is usually said to originate with the French philosopher René Descartes (1596–1650) who first argued that intangibles, such as religious faith, had no place in the physical world. Descartes is generally credited with inventing the 'mechanist' approach which finally split science and medicine from religion. Factors which were not physically demonstrable – such as inner energy – were dismissed as mere acts of faith and relegated to the world of superstition and myth. If it could not be demonstrated by science then, argued the 'enlightened' eighteenth century scientific pioneers, it did not exist.

This mechanistic separation means that illness is largely defined purely in terms of pathology, rather than in relation to the whole person and their emotional or spiritual well-being. In many older healing traditions the opposite is still true. Emotional and spiritual unrest are just as valid causes of 'dis-ease' as invading pathogens or a failure of the immune system.

In these traditions, rather than simply being regarded as a mechanical pump for the circulation, the heart, for example, is closely associated with emotional and spiritual influences. The ancient Chinese saw it as the centre of *Shen* – the spirit – while in Ayurveda – the ancient medicine of India – the heart is the home of the *atman*, the true or divine aspect of our beings. The dominance of heart disease in our culture may have less to do with excess cholesterol and rather more to do with the lack of spirituality in our society. As Ayurvedic expert David Frawley (1989), points out, the reason why heart disease is so prevalent in our society is not just a matter of bad diet and overwork: 'Many of us literally die of broken hearts or spiritual starvation.'

While traditional societies still look for spiritual causes for illness, a disharmony with surroundings or suppressed negative emotions, Western orthodox practitioners prefer to put the blame on 'stress' and offer anti-depressants.

While alleviating 'stress' – the irritant causing the basic disease – is an important aspect of healing, so too is the need to reconnect body, mind and spirit. In the last 200 years much of our human spirituality has continued to wither under the continued demands for proof, until, now the very expression 'spirit' needs some explanation. And there is nothing very new about our confusion, as Patrick Pietroni (1990) explains:

> The divide between spirit and mind is not helped by the fact that the translators of Freud translated the German word *der Siele* (soul)

as 'mind' and used the Greek work *'psyche',* meaning soul, to describe mental structure. Thus, in a cosmic Freudian slip, the discussion regarding the separation between mind and spirit is made almost impossible.

Trying to have it all

While striving for some goal or objective is a normal aspect of everyday living, the objectives need to be realistic and kept in healthy perspective. Modern western society, sadly, tends to concentrate on consumption, acquisition and success. Parents put pressure on their children to achieve high exam grades, middle-ranking executives become depressed by any perceived lack of promotional success, and 'keeping up with the Jones' – even if that means going into debt to do so – is considered quite normal. In the late Frank Muir's autobiography, *A Kentish Lad* (Muir, 1997) he talks of the advent of television and how, in the 1950s, even those who could not afford to buy or rent a set used to have a television aerial erected on their roofs to suggest to the neighbours that they could. Such behaviour would be quite laughable if it were not, sadly, true – and also as likely today as it was fifty years ago

Escaping from these social pressures and understanding what is enough for our needs – and the difference between 'need' and 'want' – is an essential aspect of avoiding excessive anxiety and stress. Being satisfied with what we *have* rather than what we *could have* can make life a great deal simpler.

The philosopher Roger Scruton (2002) talks of contemporary society having as its goal 'pleasure', which he defines as 'agitation, consumption and relentless creation of waste – both material and spiritual'. In contrast, traditional cultures and, until comparatively recently, western society, laid greater emphasis on 'happiness' – a state of being that involves 'serenity, acceptance and a quiet joy in the ordinary things'.

This sort of 'happiness' is very akin to the sort of feelings traditional kava drinkers, coca or khat chewers describe when they have imbibed their favourite herbs. Achieving this sort of happiness without the need to use artificial means must surely be a worthy goal for us all.

CHAPTER 2

Herbs, mind and mood

> . . .the plant [coca] do make them drunke and bee out of judgement; they mingle coca leaves with tabaco and chew together and goe as if they were out of their wittes . . .
>
> Nicholas Monardes in *Joyfull News out of the New Found Worlde* 1577

Herbs – in all cultures – have always been regarded as offering rather more than basic symptomatic relief for assorted physical ailments. Earlier societies thought it perfectly normal to describe herbs as 'strengthening determination', 'lifting the spirits', or to 'make the heart merry'. *Macer's Herbal,* written in the tenth century and translated into English in 1373 by John Lelamoure, describes wood betony as powerful against 'wikked sperytis' while simply looking on the common pot marigold will 'drawyth owt of ye heed wikked hirores' [draw evil humours from the head]. Drinking dandelion infusion reputedly helped encourage psychic abilities, while eyebright is still regarded by some (Ryall, 1996) as an effective herb for clearing the mind and encouraging visions.

Herbs were regularly worn in amulets both for health reasons and for more subtle mysteries: a pot marigold amulet was believed to give the wearer a vision of anyone who had robbed him while vervain was associated with fortune telling until at least the seventeenth century. Honeysuckle was supposed to bring good luck while stinging nettles could be used to repel curses.

Numerous plants were attributed with combating evil, ensuring a happy life or a power to deflect lightning strikes. Until the early years of the twentieth century in more remote country districts, sprigs of St John's wort would still be worn hidden in clothing (according to some sources under the left armpit) to ward off enchantment, the evil eye, witchcraft and even death itself. Chamomile sprinkled in the house was believed to remove curses and spells while a mullein amulet was supposed both to keep wild animals at bay and encourage love from the opposite sex.

Some of these more nebulous attributes are now known to have a basis in scientific fact. Borage was traditionally associated with courage and merriment. As John Gerard writing in 1597 reminds us, quoting an old tag, '*Ego Borago gaudia semper ago*' (I borage bring always courage) and adding that the Roman writer, Pliny, called it '*Euphrosium* because it maketh a man merrie and joyful'. A generation earlier, William Turner noted that borage 'seemeth to make men merry, if they drink of the wine that it is put into'.

Today we know that borage actually does stimulate the adrenal glands to produce more adrenaline – that fight or flight hormone again – so it can, in a sense, increase our courageousness. The plant is still used by herbalists to help lift the spirits in depressive syndromes but, as is often the case, research is limited and has yet to confirm this aspect of its activity.

Herbs can act directly on the brain: there have been reports of aromatic chemicals from essential oils travelling through the olfactory system to reach parts of the limbic system in the brain – this is a complex network of nerve pathways which in humans acts as a focus for emotions and is involved in the expression of instinct and mood.

Other remedies affect different areas (Diagram 1). According to Weiss (1988) sedatives and hypnotics attach the neopallium – the part of the brain occupied with impressions from senses other than the sense of smell. Tranquillisers, like the inhaled aromatic compounds, reach the limbic system. Neuroleptics and thymoleptics – substances which (respectively) can combat psychotic symptoms and depression – impact on the hypothalamus which is

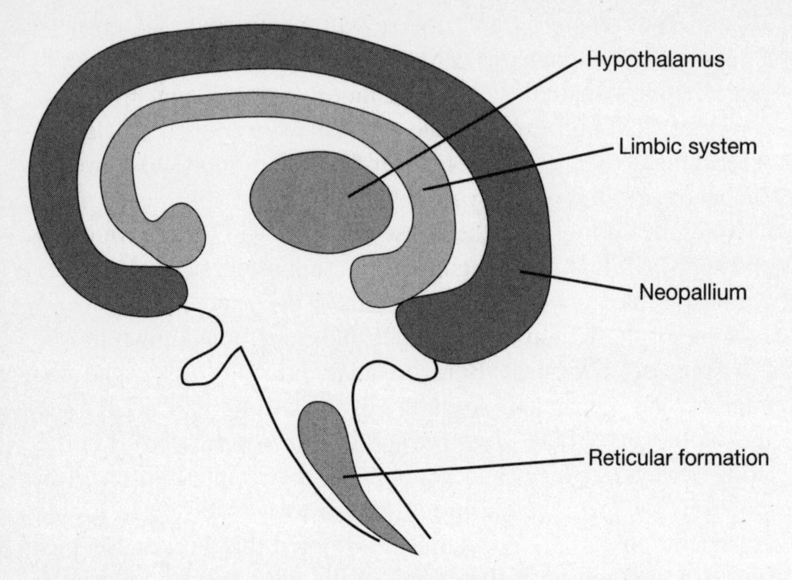

Diagram 1: Different herbal nervines affect different parts of the brain *(after Weiss, 1988)*

the part of the brain connected with emotional activity and sleep, as well as controlling body temperature, thirst, hunger and sexual function. Hypnotics and neuroleptics affect the reticular formation – an area involved with connecting motor and sensory nerves.

Potent potions

While some of these active herbs are still used in similar ways in home remedies today, others are regarded as far too powerful and potentially toxic for all but the most skilled to use. Many of our psychoactive plants have a direct impact on levels of consciousness and emotions. Deadly nightshade and its relative henbane, for example, are currently restricted to qualified practitioners and are mainly used as antispasmodics to relieve pain in severe asthma and gallbladder disorders as well as to dry excessive saliva production in Parkinson's disease. In times past both herbs were ingredients in witch's flying ointment – a mixture of hallucinogens and narcotic herbs brewed with various animal fats and rubbed under the armpits to give the illusion of flying and help the user to achieve a trance-like state.

Henbane's New World relative jimson weed, played a similar role in South American shamanic rituals and was regarded as sacred by the Aztecs. Leaves of the herb were sometimes used in sleep pillows for insomnia while, taken internally, it was used to encourage 'spirit travelling' – helping the shaman to enter the spirit world and seek to placate the angry beings causing an illness. In parts of South America jimson weed was mixed with tobacco and smoked by patients to cause a stupor which was believed to encourage healing (Schlieffer, 1973). Jimson weed is still believed by some to break spells, protect against evil spirits and is said to cure insomnia if the leaves are placed in the sufferer's shoe which must be left under the bed with the toes pointing towards the nearest wall.

Equally important in South America is peyote. This was known as the 'sacred mushroom' of the Aztecs, but is actually the bitter tops collected from a type of cactus. These are highly hallucinogenic – a series of books by Carlos Castanada describing the effects of chewing peyote achieved cult status in the 1970s. The plant contains a chemical called mescaline, which causes heightened awareness and visions, and was first noted by Western writers in the 1730s (Schlieffer, 1973). Peyote was associated with shamanic rituals and spirit travelling. Miraculous cures were associated with it and by the 1920 its use had spread to many of the southern states of North America where it was widely used by the Navaho. Peyote, also known as mescal buttons or *anhalonium*, is also a traditional remedy for asthma, gout and rheumatism although, when still used today, as in Mexico, it is mainly as a mood-enhancing hallucinogen. Possession of the herb is illegal in many countries.

Medicinal mushrooms

Mushrooms have also been appreciated by numerous cultures across the centuries both for their general medicinal use and for their psychoactive properties.

Bracket fungi which generally grow in closely packed clumps on trees or around tree stumps have been used medicinally in many parts of the world. Agaric was collected from larch trees by the second-century Greek physician, Dioscorides, and used for a lengthy list of ills, ranging from ague and 'falling sickness' (epilepsy) to consumption, asthma, digestive upsets and 'the stinging of serpents and the biting of the same'. Or as John Gerard put it in 1597: '. . .agaric maketh the body well-coloured, driveth foorth wormes, cureth agues, especially quotidians and wandering fevers, and others that are of long continuance'.

Among the more psychoactive remedies is fly agaric. Extracts were eaten by Siberian shaman to induce the trance-like state needed for spirit travelling. In South America a similar mushroom, the *nanacatl,* was known as 'flesh of the gods' and was eaten with honey to encourage a euphoric state. More recently in Western society, so-called 'magic mushrooms' have been used as hallucinogens and mind-enhancing recreational drugs – not always legally.

Ergot of rye, a parasitic fungus found on cereal crops in winter, is another strong sedative. It is a restricted poison but was once a popular choice for various hysteria states, *delirium tremens*, and also in childbirth as it has a direct effect on the uterus, encouraging contractions in the final stages of labour.

Fungi play an important part in Chinese medicine with many regarded as important energy tonics. Several species were believed by the ancient Taoists to have spiritual action to strengthen virtue and thus longevity.

Among the more exotic is 'caterpillar fungus', a parasite which grows on caterpillars of the moth *Hepialus armoricanus*, feeding on the animal and then fruiting in the spring. The traditional remedy used in China was actually a mixture of dead larva complete with their fungal parasites, although today the fungus is cultivated rather more pleasantly on a grain base.

In ancient China caterpillar fungus – known as *Dong Chong Xia Cao* which translates literally as 'winter bug, summer herb' – was kept exclusively for use by the Emperor and his household. It was always eaten with duck: five of the caterpillars would be forced into the duck's stomach and the bird was then roasted. The fungus was removed and the duck eaten twice a day for a week or more as an essential energy tonic to renew vital, inner strength.

The red bracket fungus *Ling Zhi* – now most commonly known in the West by its Japanese name '*reishi*' – was another regarded as an elixir for immortality. In Chinese writing the word *Ling* is composed of the pictograms for rain, shaman and praying which together are generally taken to mean 'spiritual potency' or a 'stirring of the soul' (Willard, 1990) while one possible interpretation of *Zhi* is 'tree fungus'. The fungus is red – a colour also associated by the ancient Chinese with the soul. In Taoist philosophy the concept of immortality was linked to following a path of virtue in harmony with the environment and greater universe and *Ling Zhi* was thus seen as strengthening the determination to follow this path and empower the soul to greater virtue and thus immortality.

Potent – but mostly illegal

Among the most potent herbs which can affect our moods or alter states of consciousness are several which today are either totally banned or restricted to use by the orthodox medical profession. The list includes Indian hemp, khat, cocaine, opium poppy, kava, and Indian snakeroot.

Indian hemp *(Cannabis sativa)*
Like opium, Indian hemp is regarded today more as a recreational drug than as a legitimate medicine. This view is starting to change, since the herb is now permitted as a painkiller and anti-

emetic in conditions such as multiple sclerosis, which respond poorly to more orthodox treatments.

Indian hemp was once recommended as a garden plant (the eighteenth- century writer, William Cobbett, in *The English Gardener*, describes it as ideal for the back of the herbaceous border) although unlicensed cultivation is now illegal. The active principle, found in a resin collected from the plant, is known as cannabinol; it stimulates the cerebrum (the most highly developed part of the brain) to produce a state of euphoria.

Indian hemp is used to produce three narcotic forms:

- marijuana (*bhang*) which is the upper part of the plant with only a little of the active resin and is generally smoked as cigarettes;
- hashish (*ganja)* prepared from selected flowers and leaves. This is rich in resin and thus more potent. It is usually taken internally and is popular in the Near East; and
- charas – the pure resin collected from careful selection of the flowering tops; this is the most potent form.

Cannabis tincture was once a popular treatment for depression; the herb produces a positive uplift in mood with a marked euphoric effect. Its use and possession is currently illegal; cultivation is similarly restricted although it can be grown under licence for medicinal or other commercial use.

Khat *(Catha edulis)*

What coca is to South America or kava to Polynesia, so khat is the African equivalent. The tree – also known as bushman's tea – grows in Africa and the Middle East and, like coca, the fresh leaves are chewed to allay hunger and combat fatigue. The bark is also used medicinally in decoctions as a nerve tonic and heart stimulant while the dried leaves are brewed for asthma and coughs.

Khat chewing is seen by many users as a harmless social activity little different from drinking coffee – it is a largely male activity, with groups resting on cushions in a relaxed atmosphere, happily sharing their khat leaves. Critics point to such adverse effects as dependency, increased sleepiness, loss of appetite and risk of psychosis, although the evidence is disputed.

Chewing khat is regarded by many as a problem for migrant communities, since importing the fresh leaves into Europe is expensive, so leisurely khat chewing gatherings are regarded as a waste of both time and money.

The plant's main constituent (cathimone) has a similar action to amphetamines – a pharmaceutical stimulant (Conway, 2001). Use of the herb is restricted in many countries.

Coca *(Erythroxylum coca)*

Chewing – or rather sucking – the leaves of the coca tree is a traditional social activity in many parts of Peru, Bolivia and Colombia. Friends gather to sit and share their leaves at times of trouble or when they have problems to discuss. Others chew coca mid morning or in the afternoon – much as we in Europe would take a coffee or tea break. Chewing the dry leaves releases the potent alkaloids, including cocaine, which the plant contains. These have a bitter taste, so lime or powdered ash is sometimes added to counteract the unpleasant flavour. Coca's alkaloids have a stimulating effect on the central nervous system; the leaves were traditionally taken by the Incas on long journeys to help combat hunger and fatigue.

The herb has been used in South America since at least 3000BC – remains of the leaves have been found in ancient tombs. It was known as the 'divine plant' by the Incas who extensively cultivated the herb from as early as the twelfth century – reputedly they regarded it as more valuable than gold. Its use was first noted by Europeans in the early sixteenth century and by 1569 Catholic bishops had condemned chewing coca leaves as creating 'an illusion of the devil' (Madge, 2001).

The plant was brought to England in the 1840s and research in Germany and Austria in the 1850s first isolated and identified its potent alkaloids. By the 1860s cocaine had started to be used as a local anaesthetic – notably by the Austrian surgeon Karl Koller, who used it in eye operations. In South America the leaves are still made into an ointment in folk medicine to relieve pain, while infusions are also given for gastric upsets, altitude sickness, rheumatism and malaria.

At one time the leaves were regarded as an innocent remedy to combat fatigue – so much so that they were once combined with caffeine-rich kola nuts to create a restorative drink called Coca-Cola (which, of course, no longer contains either coca or kola). Today, in Europe and North America, however, coca tends to be regarded as a potent and addictive stimulant.

The effect of chewing the leaves is reputedly quite mild and tonifying – just enough to relieve exhaustion and lift the spirits. If the powdered extract is snorted (as happens in recreational drug taking) it has a much more dramatic effect giving a euphoric high which can last for up to an hour. Users feel self-confident with enhanced sensory perception. In this form it can be highly addictive and long-term use may lead to severe depression. Its use and possession is illegal.

Opium poppy *(Papaver somniferum)*

The opium poppy provides us with the drug morphine as well as highly addictive heroin – traffic in which is associated with so much organised crime. To an earlier generation tincture of opium was 'laudanum', an apparently calming and anti-depressive remedy which many thousands of Victorian ladies – including it is said Queen Victoria – took perhaps rather too regularly.

The noted German herbalist, Rudolf Weiss (1988) puts opium at the top of his scale of herbal remedies for nervous disorders with milder herbs such as valerian and lemon balm at the bottom, and St John's wort somewhere in between. He argues that the herb should still be valued as an effective remedy for depression particularly in difficult or persistent cases where addiction is not likely to be a problem. Weiss suggests a standard dose of five drops of opium tincture three times a day, increasing gradually to twenty drops, before being reduced and withdrawn as the patient recovers. He also argues that at least two-thirds of the cases of severe depression can be successfully treated with this sort of opium therapy and questions why the approach has fallen so far from favour among modern practitioners.

According to Rudolf Weiss, very small doss of opium tincture can be effective for depression associated with the menopause – one reason why it was so popular among our middle-aged Victorian ancestresses – as well as for depression in the elderly. He recommends adding just one part of opium tincture to twenty parts of valerian tincture and ten parts of lily-of-the-valley tincture, with the mixture given in a dose of just ten drops so that the opium content is thus minimal.

***Kava** (Piper methysticum)*

One of the latest herbs to join the lists of those banned or restricted has been kava. The herb has been used in rites and ceremonies since well before Dutch explorers such as Le Maire and Schouten first described its use in 1616. Captain Cook (1777) noted during his visit to the Society Islands, that:

> Sometimes they [the natives] chew this root in their mouths as Europeans do tobacco, and swallow their spittle; and sometimes I have seen them eat it wholly. At Ulieta they cultivate great quantities of this plant . . . making a liquor from a plant in the same manner as here mentioned.

Kava is still used in formal ceremonies, such as welcoming royalty or high-ranking honoured guests; it is drunk at meetings of village elders and visiting chiefs; it may be drunk at a social gathering most usually to seal a contract or during trading negotiations; and it can also be drunk as part of religious rites – such as during ancestor worship rituals in pre-Christian Fiji. Commonly the herb is also just consumed, rather like coffee or wine, as a regular evening beverage. Lebot *et al.* (1997) describe various kava-drinking practices in village gatherings and in the kava-bars – variously named *sakau* bars or *nakamal* – which are found in the more westernised islands.

Alcohol was unknown in the various Pacific Islands until the arrival of Europeans, and kava took its place as a relaxing drink which encouraged a euphoric state of mind and oiled social interactions. Central to the more formalised ceremonial are the kava bowl (known as *tano'a* in Tongan or *tanoa* in Fijian), the strainer and the cup along with the kava root stock and water. The herb was traditionally chewed, typically by young girls or men, before being placed in the traditional bowl, half-filled with cold water. A fibrous strainer usually made from hibiscus bark (*H. tilitaceus*) was then laid on the mixture and the soaked kava systematically collected and squeezed. Cups of kava were then filled and distributed in strict order of social status: honoured guests followed by the most senior chief and so on down the hierarchy.

The plant is generally drunk in the evenings often in silence: on the island of Tanna (Lindstrom, 1981) they believe that too much noise may 'kill the kava' and in order to appreciate its psychoactive effects drinkers prefer silence, dusk and firelight to '*harem singsing blong kava*' (listen to the song of the kava). The herb is generally taken before the evening meal as a full stomach can reduce the appreciation of its psychoactive properties and the evening meal is always small as the herb acts as an appetite suppressant and over-eating after kava can lead to nausea.

As well as its ritual use, the root extract is given in the South Seas for genital infections, menstrual syndromes, headaches, general debility, colds and chills, chest pains, or as a tonic. The plant is antiseptic, will ease spasmodic cramps and encourages urination so can be helpful for urinary tract problems such as cystitis. Reports of kava as a remedy for urinary ailments first appeared in the West in 1818 (Whistler, 1992) and the herb was introduced into Europe as a medicinal remedy in the 1850s – imported primarily as a cure for gonorrhoea and urinary tract problems.

Kava numbs the mouth and tongue and is mildly paralysing, while creating a clear-minded state in which the drinker cannot be annoyed. It is an effective soporific widely used for sleep problems. In recent years kava has achieved a worldwide reputation as a nerve relaxant to dispel inhibitions and anxieties. As such it has almost achieved recreational drug status in parts of the West with kava-based remedies variously recommended for stress, anxiety, insomnia, panic attacks, headaches, back pains, depression, fatigue, muscle pains, or menstrual upsets – as well as being heavily promoted as 'perfect for people who feel awkward at parties', or 'ideal when everyday worries interfere with social interactions'.

Kava's popularity led to widespread marketing of highly concentrated extracts with excessive doses consumed in self-medication by those who had taken the marketing hype rather too much to heart. Towards the end of 2001 there were reports from Germany and Switzerland of a growing number of cases of liver damage linked to the herb which led UK health food producers to agree to a voluntary withdrawal of the remedy from their shelves. The German drugs regulatory authority, BfArm, collected thirty case reports of liver damage among kava takers. These cases ranged from four instances of increased liver enzyme production and five of gall bladder inflammation to five instances of liver failure, including one fatality. Only three of the patients were not also taking additional medication, so blaming kava without investigating what also was being swallowed could be regarded as a little blinkered.

In the three cases of liver transplantation following liver failure, cited in the report, all involved high kava doses – as much as 480 mg daily – for long periods. The official daily dose of kava, recommended in Germany's Commission E monographs – widely regarded as one of the world's most authoritative sources on the therapeutics of medicinal plants – is 60–120 mg of kavalactones (the active chemicals within the plant) daily. There have also been a handful of adverse reports in the UK: one (Escher *et al.*, 2001) involved a fifty-year-old man who developed jaundice caused by hepatitis after taking the equivalent of 210–280 mg of kavalactones daily.

Over the past forty years there have been numerous studies on the properties of kava's active group of constituents, known

Table 2: Relative analgesic effect

	Dosage required for equivalent effect (mg/kg)
Morphine	002.5
Dimethylaminophenazone	100.0
Kavalactones	
Dihydrokavain (DHK)	120.0
Dihydromethysticin (DHM)	120.0
Aspirin	200.0

(Source: Lebot et al., 1997, adapted from Hänsel, 1968)

kavalactones. One important constituent, dihydromethysticin (DHM), can significantly enhance the effect of conventional barbiturates (Hänsel, 1968) while several studies have also looked at the different analgesic properties of the kavalactones; while these are much less than such potent drugs as morphine, they are rather more significant that aspirin (Table 2)

Studies (Singh, 1983) suggest that kava has a direct effect on the contractibility of skeletal muscle, rather like some local anaesthetics, as well as probably some action on the central nervous system rather like barbiturates and tranquillisers. Other actions of kavalactones confirmed over the years include anti-bacterial and anti-fungal action. Kava extracts can also suppress the release of glutamates by brain cells, which could thus act as a preventative for strokes, and also have blood-thinning properties (Gleitz *et al.*, 1996; 1997) rather like aspirin and ginkgo.

In clinical trials kava has been shown to improve sleep patterns, reduce anxiety levels, improve concentration, and enhance the activity of a number of commonly used pharmaceutical drugs (Furgiuele *et al.*, 1965; Johnson *et al.*, 1991; Lehmann, *et al.*, 1996; Scholing and Clausen, 1977; Woelk *et al.*, 1993). In a project lasting for more six months and involving 100 patients (Volz and Kieser, 1997) given either a 300mg dose of kava or placebo. The kava patients showed significant and sustained improvements in anxiety levels. Kava has also been shown to be helpful for menopausal emotional upsets, epilepsy and depression (see Mills and Bone, 2000 for a full review).

Despite this impressive litany, excessive use of kava concentrates have persuaded many regulatory bodies to ban kava and it is no longer available in the UK or Germany.

Indian snakeroot *(Rauwolfia serpentina)*

Until the 1960s, Indian snakeroot was one of the herbalist's most commonly used remedies for reducing high blood pressure and treating psychiatric and nervous problems. The herb acts on the limbic system of the brain and in medium doses, this reduces levels of catecholamines and noradrenaline which in turn leads to relaxation of the peripheral blood vessels and thus a lowering of blood-pressure levels.

In larger doses Indian snakeroot acts as a neuroleptic capable of influencing psychotic symptoms, delusions and hallucinations. It was thus once the herb of choice for treating schizophrenia. However, in such high doses it can lead to symptoms of parkinsonism with tremors of the hands and changes in brain chemistry.

In very low doses the herb has a tranquillising effect and can relieve anxiety and tension helping to normalise outlook and emotional balance. It was often used in combination with valerian (two parts valerian to one part Indian snakeroot). In the UK the herb is now severely restricted and is available only on prescription from registered medical practitioners, so it is rarely used.

In traditional Indian medicine the herb – variously known as *chota chund, chandrabhaga, chundrika* and by dozens of other local dialect names – is used as a remedy for insomnia, fevers, epilepsy and various nervous disorders. It is also given as a calming remedy in childbirth.

CHAPTER 3

Discovering herbal alternatives

> The presenting disease is readily identified but it tends to be regarded as an entity in its own right, instead of being, as in fact it is, merely the ultimate and physical manifestation of a state of imbalance affecting the total energy system.
>
> Ian Pearce, in the *Gate of Healing, 1973*

In recent years the importance of stress in triggering disease has become more widely accepted but – as discussed in Chapter 1 – emotional factors, too, play a part. Traditional therapies still make this important association. In Chinese medicine, for example, each major body organ is associated with a particular emotion: the liver links with anger, the kidneys with fear, the lungs with grief. These associations are not unfamiliar: we all know how fear can send us trotting to spend yet another penny as the urinary system appears to go into overdrive, while even in the West we associate feeling 'liverish' with irritability and bad temper. Commonly, too, those suffering a bereavement succumb to some sort of lung problem – bronchitis or asthma in the recently widowed is extremely common.

The late Ian Pearce, renowned for his pioneering cancer treatments, stressed this fundamental connection in his approach to both diagnosis and therapeutics arguing that: 'We create our own health, just as we create our own diseases' (1983). He would point out that modern medication, while alleviating symptoms, did not always cure the underlying dis-ease. One of his examples was pneumonia which in the days before antibiotics would reach a 'crisis' on the eighth day, when patients would emerge from their delirium or succumb to the disease. Modern drugs bring down temperature and appear to effect a 'cure' within thirty-six hours – yet the chest is still not clear until the eighth day, just as in the pre-antibiotic days.

Pearce, a GP for most of his working life, maintained that the illnesses of around 75per cent of his patients were caused by stresses that they could not control. 'Stress,' he said, 'is a state of mind. We create it out of the way we respond to things around us.'

Equally, psychological problems may be related to some sort of physical imbalance. The Chinese, as we have seen, link the heart with the spirit. They also connect it with an emotion – usually translated as 'joy' which seems to westerners a very positive concept unlikely to led to ill heath. It is better regarded as a form of manic or inappropriate behaviour, which in such a rigidly hierarchical society as Imperial China, would have had far more negative connotations. Surprisingly frequently, people who seem to maintain odd tangential conversations making inappropriate remarks with no sense of continuity in their conversation, seem to suffer from some sort of heart problem or have raised blood pressure.

Orthodox practitioners often dismiss illnesses as 'psychosomatic' – a problem with the mind (*psyche*) leading to body (*soma*) disorders – and prescribe anti-depressants. But this is simply to reinforce the mechanistic divide between body, mind and spirit. If a person thinks they are ill, then they are ill and simply focusing on medical pathology will do little to solve the underlying problems. Equally, the physical illness may be the result of a complex mesh of emotional and spiritual problems finally manifesting as a physical disorder. As most of us know only too well, if we're happy we're generally well, but if we're not or dislike our jobs we're far more likely to take days off due to sickness – real or imaginary.

If we accept that illness is not always simply a physical

affliction then the way that we treat those disorders needs to change. If the physical illness arises from some emotional imbalance or dysfunctional lifestyle, then all the medication in the world is not going to solve the problem.

Almost any illness may have causal factors which include stress, psychological or emotional problems, and sufferers should always seek to assess the impact of these on their dis-ease. The rest of this chapter is devoted to some of the more commonly stress-related disorders listed alphabetically. In each case suggestions are given for suitable herbal approaches to treatment. Full details of the more important plants mentioned to combat stress, tension or depression can be found in Chapter 4. As always, accurate diagnosis is essential and it is important to seek professional help for any long-standing condition or where unusual symptoms persist for more than a few days.

Allergies, hyperactivity and auto-immune disorders

Allergies are increasingly common in our highly stressed environment. More children suffer from peanut allergy, asthma or eczema than ever before and clearly there are environmental and dietary factors involved in this polluted world of ours. An allergy is simply an abnormally sensitive reaction to a substance or the environment. The ‘allergens’ causing the problem can be many and varied: pollen, milk, cleaning fluids, metal, wheat, house dust, or animal hair for example. The allergic response can range from the itching eyes and running nose familiar in hayfever to skin rashes or joint pains.

An exacerbation in the allergic response often coincides with a stressful period: teenage hay fever sufferers are usually worse at exam times while eczema will flare into unsightly rashes just before the crucial job interview. One reason is that the allergen itself is acting as a stress on the body’s normal function so that when additional problems appear, in the form of family worries or work pressure, the combined stresses cause a manifold increase in the usual allergic reactions.

Identifying and avoiding the primary allergens causing the stress are clearly important. Herbal treatment is likely to include anti-allergy remedies to help reduce sensitivity, anti-stress herbs and specific remedies to relieve the relevant symptoms. These may be combined with relaxing regimes – such as deep breathing or simple yoga exercises – to help calm the sufferer, as well as with nutritional advice to help balance diet and avoid excessive intake of the suspect allergens.

Typical anti-allergy remedies include:

- stinging nettles taken in teas
- chamomile used in teas, steam inhalations or essential oils
- garlic best used regularly in cooking, and
- *Ma Huang* – also known as ephedra and the source of the drug ephedrine – a potent remedy which is restricted in the UK to professional practitioners.

These anti-allergenic remedies could be combined with relaxing herbs such as valerian or Siberian ginseng to help increase the body's ability to deal with stress.

Hyperactivity in children is also often associated with allergies and is especially common in asthma and eczema sufferers. Over-active children will – sooner or later – almost inevitably have over-stressed parents with bad tempers all round. Food colourants, especially tartrazine and 'sunshine yellow', are often to blame for such abnormal behaviour while too many excessively sweet snacks and soft drinks simply add to the imbalance.

Chinese medicine sees hyperactivity as a form of excessive liver energy to be treated with cooling remedies, notably self-heal. Chamomile is also particularly good for such children – 500 ml of strained infusion can be added to bath water so that the sufferer inhales the soothing and anti-allergenic compounds produced in the steam. Linden is another suitably calming remedy while agrimony is always worth considering in cases of food allergy as it helps to strengthen and desensitise the system.

Auto-immune diseases, such as psoriasis, ulcerative colitis and rheumatoid arthritis, occur when the body attacks itself with its own defence mechanism and starts to destroy or damage healthy tissue. The cause is still poorly understood but stress and emotional factors appear to play a part. These sorts of conditions are often worse when external stresses increase, while the initial trigger is sometimes a major emotional trauma. I once had a patient, a professional musician, whose psoriasis had started when her mother died suddenly; the skin condition flared up whenever there was a particularly important performance pending. Another, suffering from rheumatoid arthritis, was always rather worse on the days before her husband had to go away on a business trip – increasing his feelings of guilt at leaving her and emphasising her dependence.

Symptom-specific remedies are an important part of treatment but flower essences (such as Dr Bach's remedies detailed below) can often help to restore emotional balance and help sufferers to understand any underlying causes affecting their condition.

Allergies, hyperactivity and – especially – auto-immune problems really need professional help to identify and minimise causal factors with appropriate remedies.

Anxiety

Anxiety is one of those vague terms which can mean many different things to different people. All of us feel some degree of anxiety at times – especially before an exam or when loved ones are late coming home – but anxiety only becomes a medical problem when it starts to interfere with everyday life and activities.

A label of 'anxiety' can cover worry, mild depression, constant feelings of tension and an inability to relax. Anxiety can also be associated with a failure to cope with 'stress' and is a characteristic of all psychiatric disorders. Typical symptoms can include a dry mouth and increased sweating, fainting, rapid heartbeat or shortness of breath.

Anxiety can also be classified as a single ailment in 'anxiety neurosis'. This disorder can include recurrent panic attacks, which may last from a few minutes to an hour or two. Sufferers may experience a subjective sense of terror for no apparent reason or a dread of some nameless catastrophe which interferes with normal, rational behaviour. The attack is likely to be accompanied by increased heart rate or palpitations, a fine tremor in the hands, possible chest pains, 'butterflies in the stomach', sweating, nausea and dizziness to varying degrees. The panic attack may also include breathing problems or hyperventilation which generally increase the sense of panic and impending doom.

Anxiety-like symptoms can also occur with other physical ailments so any chronic or persistent problems need professional investigation. Palpitations, chest pains and breathing difficulties, for example, are associated with heart disorders, such as angina pectoris, while nervousness, irritability, sweating and palpitations are among the symptoms of an over-active thyroid gland.

Anxiety is always helped by talking over the problem with a wise counsellor, but herbs can also play a part, both for the minor transient anxiousness we all feel from time to time, and the more severe forms of the condition which can lead to debilitating panic attacks.

Readily available herbs for use in calming teas at home include passion flower, chamomile, linden, skullcap, motherwort, wood betony, and wild lettuce. These herbs can be combined as need be to make pleasant-tasting and effective remedies. Equal parts of motherwort, lemon balm and skullcap, for example, will make a suitably broad spectrum and soothing brew.

Time spent making tea is always an important part of the therapeutic process when using herbal remedies. It can be particularly helpful whenever stress is a factor forcing us to find time to make the brew, sit quietly and sip the remedy. For those with hectic lifestyles the half-hour or so this can take provides an important punctuation mark in the day – a time to sit, relax and do absolutely nothing.

For those prone to panic attacks a dropper bottle containing good quality tinctures of any of these relaxing herbs makes a useful standby bringing quick relief of symptoms in a moderately convenient form; put three to five drops on the tongue as often need be. Rose tincture can also be especially helpful for panic attacks as can Dr Bach's Rescue Remedy.

Valerian is a popular option widely available as capsules or tablets from health food shops – a useful option as the flavour is not to everyone's taste. Valerian is sometimes described as 'nature's tranquilliser', a calming and relaxing remedy which sedates without causing drowsiness.

Until recently, when concerns over toxicity led to restrictions in its sale, kava was one of the more popular over-the-counter options for anxiety problems – with numerous enthusiastic trials (Medi-Herb, 1996) reporting significant reduction in anxiety levels over long time scales.

Depression

While we all tend to feel down from time to time, clinical depression is a debilitating illness that needs professional help. This should preferably include counselling and psychiatric help rather than simply repeat prescriptions of anti-depressant drugs which can have side-effects and will not necessarily provide a long-term cure.

Depression is often associated with withdrawal – avoiding normal social activities or lacking the energy even to get out of bed in the morning. As well as this 'closing down' of normal emotional activity there can be a physical closing down too: depressives, for example, often suffer from constipation – a physical manifestation of their internal focus.

Interestingly, in the traditional Galenic medicine of western Europe – practised from Roman times until the seventeenth century – depression was regarded as 'melancholia' and was considered to be the result of too much 'black bile' in the system. Black bile was regarded as one of the four humours (along with blood, phlegm and yellow bile) which the body contained and whose balance was essential for good health.

An excess of black bile (i.e. melancholia) would be treated with strong purgatives and digestive remedies to cleanse the system. A surviving prescription written by William Harvey (1578–1657), who first described the circulation of the blood, for the essayist John Aubrey in 1655, well demonstrates the approach with a highly cathartic brew containing: rhubarb root, agaric, black hellebore, dates and senna, curiously designed to put the patient in a more uplifting mood.

Modern herbalists prefer less dramatic treatments using a mixture of relaxing herbs to ease stress and tension and specifics to ease particular symptoms as well as those which have a positive effect on lifting the spirits. Typical relaxing remedies could be passion flower, lemon balm, skullcap or chamomile. Motherwort could be added if palpitations are a problem or black cohosh if the mood change is linked to menstrual irregularities. Remedies in the more uplifting or 'thymoleptic' category include damiana, black cohosh, wild oats and wood betony. Wild oats work particularly well in combination with damiana and vervain. Sometimes more active stimulation is needed and herbs like Korean ginseng, rosemary, guarana and even kola – a rich source of caffeine – can sometimes help to refuel energy levels.

Adding a digestive stimulant – such as dandelion root, holy thistle or liquorice – to the remedy can also help improve general well-being. A modern herbal approach thus involves countering any physical exhaustion and debility, which may be contributing to the problem, stimulating the digestive system if need be, and using herbs to strengthen the nervous system.

St John's wort, traditionally used by herbalists to strengthen and repair the nervous system, has received its fair share of publicity in recent years as an effective anti-depressant. In Germany it has become the remedy of choice in mild cases, preferred by many orthodox doctors to more conventional pharmaceutical drugs. Inevitably there has been a downside with a range of side-effects reported where patients take high doses for long periods (see Chapter 4). These criticisms are not always justified but use of the herb has been restricted in some countries as a result. St John's wort is a valuable anti-depressant remedy in mild and moderately severe cases and as long as it is used in moderation for short periods is as safe as any other drug.

Depression in the elderly can be linked to poor cerebral circulation leading to forgetfulness and apparent signs of dementia. Ginkgo, skullcap, and wood betony can be especially helpful in such cases.

In traditional Chinese medicine depression is generally seen as a symptom of spleen imbalance with the spleen's associated emotion – worry – interfering with the organ's physical role (as defined in traditional Chinese medicine) of transporting nutrients and water through the body. This is then believed to lead to *Qi* (vital energy) stagnation with symptoms of depression, poor appetite, restless sleep, forgetfulness and palpitations. Ayurvedic medicine also sees chronic depression – as with other mental problems – as a whole-body syndrome which may be associated with spiritual factors leading to apathy, inertia and delusion. Treatment involves meditation and yoga as well as dietary changes and the use of *sattvic* herbs which help to encourage mental clarity, light, perception, intelligence and harmony. These include *shatavari*, *jatamansi, jati* (jasmine), and basil.

Emotional upsets

Modern medicine tends to leave emotional problems to psychologists and counsellors but, as discussed earlier, they can have a very real impact on physical wellbeing. Herbs can have a significant effect on the mind and emotions in ways which we are only beginning to understand. As already noted, there have been reports of aromatic chemicals from essential oils travelling through the olfactory system to reach parts of the limbic centre in the brain. Aromatherapy tends to be regarded in the UK as a massage-based technique, but purists in mainland Europe prefer to think of it – as the name implies – as a therapy associated with smells. Smelling certain oils can be stimulating and uplifting, while others have a more soothing and relaxing effect. Using oils in diffusers to scent rooms or adding a few drops to bath water are easy ways to influence the emotions. Among the many herb oils that can be used in this way are chamomile, lavender, marjoram, melissa (lemon balm) and neroli. Useful oils for treating nervous problems are summarised in Table 3.

Chinese tradition also closely links the emotions to specific body organs with imbalance in the physical body blamed for emotional lability and upsets. The five main organs of traditional Chinese medicine (TCM) –lungs, liver, heart, kidneys and spleen – are each linked to a specific emotion: grief, anger, manic joy, fear, and worry, respectively. The organs and emotions are mutually inter-dependent so that an excess of worry, for example, may lead to digestive upsets while liver imbalance could make the sufferer irritable and angry.

In Ayurvedic medicine, too, it is impossible to separate emotional well-being from the whole person and herbs can be used to strengthen and normalise the various energy centres or *chakras* which are linked to the mind and behaviour. These centres are believed to run in a line from the crown of the head to the base of

Table 3: Some useful essential oils

Category	Oils
Anxiety	benzoin, chamomile, clary sage, jasmine, lavender, marjoram, melissa, neroli, rose, sandalwood, ylang ylang
Depression	basil, chamomile, clary sage, lavender, melissa, rose, sandalwood, ylang ylang
Mental fatigue	basil, rosemary, thyme
Stress	benzoin, chamomile, clary sage, jasmine, lavender, marjoram, melissa, neroli, rose, sandalwood

the spine (the root *chakra*). Each is associated with particular body organs:

- root *chakra* – womb in women and prostate gland in men
- splenic *chakr*a – testes and ovaries
- navel *chakra* – liver and adrenal glands
- heart centre – the thymus gland and heart
- throat *chakra* – thyroid glands
- brow *chakra* – pituitary gland
- crown *chakra* – pineal gland

as well as having an emotional dimension.

The navel *chakra*, for example, is linked to the more negative emotions like fear and anger, the throat *chakra* is linked by some with envy, while the heart *chakra* is connected with more positive feelings of love and compassion. Emotional imbalance can thus affect the energy flow through the *chakras* which in turn is linked to weakness in the associated body organs.

Herbs can also be used to strengthen the *chakras*. The familiar culinary herb basil, for example, is believed to reinforce the root, splenic and navel *chakras*, while plants like lavender and elecampane are said to act on the crown *chakra*. Using these types of herbs in conjunction with remedies for physical complaints can be very effective.

Ayurveda also relates emotional or mental problems to imbalance in the *gunas* – the three essential qualities of matter [*sattva* (clarity), *rajas* (action) and *tamas* (desire)] and the *tri-doshas* (three humours) which as in western Galenic theory need to be kept in balance to maintain health. Nerve impulses themselves belong to the *vata* or wind humour, so *vata* disorders always involve some sort of weakness or hypersensitivity in the nervous system and are called *vatavyadhi* or *vata* diseases.

As well as using appropriate herbs, Ayurveda also recommends a variety of gem treatments for energy and emotional imbalances. This generally simply means wearing a ring or other jewel with the appropriate stone. Green stones – emerald, jade and peridot – are preferred for nervous function and nerve pains while yellow stones, such as topaz and citrine, can help strengthen the nerves and ease emotional problems associated with hormonal imbalance as at the menopause. Pearl and silver are linked to the moon and are believed to be calming and nurturing for the mind and emotions, while gold is stimulating and restorative for the nerves.

Like their Chinese and Ayurvedic counterparts, western herbalists regard emotions as closely intertwined with physical well-being. Motherwort, mugwort and wood betony, for example, are particularly suitable for menopausal emotional problems; lemon balm and chamomile for sadness and worry, or rose-petal tea for feeling neglected and unloved.

The flower remedies – discovered initially by Dr Edward Bach in the 1930s – can be particularly helpful to ease specific emotional states. There are three main types on the market: Bach Flower Remedies, Flower Essence Society Quintessentials, which originate from California, and Australian Bush Flower Essences.

Flower essences are essentially the 'dew' collected from certain flowers preserved in brandy. This basic essence is believed to incorporate some unseen energy from the flower which imbues the remedy with healing properties. They should be further diluted in water before being taken in drop doses. By this stage flower essences are in homoeopathic dilution and many orthodox practitioners are sceptical of their action but such remedies can be extremely helpful for a great many people and are worth trying.

It is interesting to compare the various remedies: Dr Bach's healers were fewer and focused on simple emotional concepts such as self-hatred, guilt or fear of the unknown. Those developed more recently feature complex specific emotional states – such as difficulties with relationships, problems with commitment, or with unresolved conflicts concerning father figures – which perhaps reflect the more introspective nature of our society.

While many people find these sorts of remedies helpful, others

Table 4: Some useful essential oils

Remedy	Dr Bach's suggested use
Agrimony	For those who suffer mental torture behind a 'brave face'
Aspen	For vague fears of an unknown origin
Beech	For critical intolerance of others
Centaury	For the weak-willed
Cerato	For those who doubt their own judgement and seek advice of others
Cherry Plum	For fears of mental collapse
Chestnut Bud	For a refusal to learn from past mistakes
Chicory	For possessiveness and selfishness
Clematis	For the inattentive and dreamy escapist
Crab Apple	A cleansing remedy for those who feel unclean or ashamed
Elm	For those temporarily overcome by feelings of inadequacy
Gentian	For the despondent and easily discouraged
Gorse	For hopelessness and despair
Heather	For the self-centred obsessed with their own troubles
Holly	For those who are jealous, angry or feel hatred for others
Honeysuckle	For home sickness and nostalgia
Hornbeam	For 'Monday morning feelings' and procrastination
Impatiens	For the impatient
Larch	For those who lack confidence
Mimulus	For fear of known things
Mustard	For deep gloom and severe depression
Oak	For those who struggle on against adversity
Olive	For complete exhaustion
Pine	For guilt feelings and self-blame
Red Chestnut	For excessive fear for others, especially loved ones
Rock Rose	For extreme terror
Rock Water	For the self-repressed who overwork and deny themselves any relaxation
Scleranthus	For uncertainty and indecision
Star of Bethlehem	For shock
Sweet Chestnut	For extreme anguish; the limit of endurance
Vervain	For tenseness, over-enthusiasm and over-effort
Vine	For the dominating and inflexible
Walnut	Provides protection at times of change such as the menopause or during other major life stage transitions
Water Violet	For the proud and reserved

Table 4: Continued

Remedy	Dr Bach's suggested use
White Chestnut	For mental anguish and persistent nagging worries
Wild Oat	For uncertainty about which path to take; an aid to decision taking
Wild Rose	For the apathetic who lack ambition
Willow	For the resentful and bitter who are fond of saying 'not fair'

argue that they are little more than placebos. Scientific studies fail to identify anything tangible in the remedies beyond a little brandy. However, they can be effective: flower essences often provide effective remedies for minor daily upsets that are both safe and convenient.

Details of Dr Edward Bach's thirty-eight healing remedies are listed in Table 4. Having chosen a suitable selection of remedies put four drops of each into a 10 ml dropper bottle and then fill this with spring water. Drop doses of the remedy can then be taken on the tongue as often as required.

The California-based Flower Essence Society (FES) supplies around 100 healing essences – sold as 'Quintessentials' – that are based mostly on New World plants. The organisation was formed in the 1970s and its essences have a significant following in the USA, although they are less common in Europe. A selection of relevant remedies is listed in Table 5. Full listings are included in a number of books (see Kaminski,1998; McIntyre 1996). The FES remedies can be taken in the same way as Dr Bach's.

The Australian Bush Essences, like the FES series, are a comparatively new development but are becoming more familiar in Europe. There are around sixty of them, based on native Australian plants, and they can be taken in the same way as Dr Bach's Remedies. A full list is included in McIntyre (1996). Table 6 lists some relevant suggestions.

Table 5: FES Quintessentials

Remedy	Recommended use
Aloe vera	For those creative people who have over-extended themselves and feel 'burnt out' or exhausted
Angelica	For those who feel spiritually bereft and isolated; over-focused on the materialist world
Blackberry	For those lacking the will and energy to carry ideas into action
Buttercup	For those lacking self-worth
California pitcher plant	For those who feel weak or lacking in vitality
California poppy	For those lacking a solid inner life or who seek superficial spirituality through drugs
California wild rose	For those lacking enthusiasm who feel withdrawn and alienated from others.
Cayenne	For those who feel sluggish and uninspired; who are resistant to change and in a period of stagnation
Chaparral	For those overwhelmed by the modern world; it helps to protect, cleanse and combat drug addiction
Corn	For those who feel confined urban environments to be disorientating and stressful and who need help to maintain spirituality
Dandelion	For those who try to cram too much into their lives leaving no time for rest and relaxation; for over-striving
Dill	For those who feel overwhelmed and overstimulated by modern life
Dogwood	For physical tension and repressed emotions
Filaree	For those too preoccupied with details and the minutiae of life; an inability to gain a wider perspective
Fuchsia	For repressed emotions, especially anger and grief
Garlic	For those easily influenced by others, who feel weak and prone to low vitality
Hound's tongue	For over-preoccupation with the material world
Indian paintbrush	For the highly creative who lose touch with the physical world and need grounding
Indian pink	For busy people who find it difficult to focus on the still centre within
Iris	For lack of inspiration or creativity
Lady's slipper	For those unable to draw on their inner wisdom and strength to provide energy for day-to-day needs

Table 5: Continued

Remedy	Recommended use
Larkspur	For those in positions of responsibility who feel overburdened with a sense of duty
Madia	For those whose energy is easily dissipated; who feel distracted, dull and listless
Mallow	For those who feel blocked emotionally
Morning glory	For burning the candle at both ends – erratic eating and sleeping patterns which deplete energy reserves
Nasturtium	For intellectuals who neglect their emotional and physical needs, who are overly 'dry'
Pomegranate	For women finding it difficult to balance family and career demands
Rabbitbrush	For those caught up in details and events who cannot see the wood for the trees
Scarlet monkeyflower	For those who fear their intense emotions and suppress them leading to tension and inner pressure
Scotch broom	For those who feel depressed and weighed down about about their lives
Tansy	For those who feel sluggish or lethargic, indecisive or indifferent tending to procrastinate
Trillium	For those over-preoccupied with possessions and power; for excessive ambition and materialism
Yerba Santa	For unresolved or repressed emotions especially melancholy and grief
Zinnia	For those who lack humour and repress their inner child; who take life too seriously

Fatigue and lack of energy

Constant tiredness is one of the most common complaints that any western practitioner hears from his or her patients. Part of the problem is undoubtedly our over-stressed and over-polluted society, foods produced by intensive farming which offer inadequate nutrition, and lifestyle demands that lead people to believe they 'can have it all'.

Table 6: Australian Bush Flower Essences

Remedy	Recommended use
Australian Bluebell	For the insecure who regard possessions as a safety net; greedy and fearful of losing what they have
Black-eyed Susan	For those constantly rushing around, over-worked and stressed who find relaxation difficult
Bush gardenia	For those preoccupied with their own lives, interests and careers who take others around them for granted
Bush iris	For preoccupation with material life and a lack of belief or spirituality
Crowea	For those who feel uncentred, lacking energy and vitality
Five corners	For lacking self-worth
Hibbertia	For perfectionists constantly seeking self-improvement and addicted to acquiring knowledge
Isopogon	For those cut off from their emotions who are ruled by their heads
Jacaranda	For ditherers, lacking focus and dissipating energy in aimless activity
Little flannel flower	For over-seriousness, lacking humour
Macrocarpa	For those who have over-extended themselves, suffering from stress or are burnt-out
Mint bush	For those facing major challenges in their lives
Old man banksia	For lethargy, lack of energy and enthusiasm
Paw paw	For those who feel over-burdened with problems and information
Red grevillea	For those in a rut who cannot break the cycle of dependency and who lack the will to change
Silver princess	For those at a cross roads in their lives, unsure of which direction to take.
Sturt desert pea	For unresolved and repressed emotions – especially grief and melancholy
Swamp banskia	For energetic people who run out of steam generally due to stress or overwork
Tall yellow top	For the unloved and lonely who feel cut off from their roots and true feelings
Yellow cowslip orchid	For the intellectuals, judgemental and critical who deny their own emotional needs

Many sufferers expect a 'quick fix' cure and are unwilling to change their eating or living habits to allow for more relaxation and shorter working hours. Herbal stimulants are, of course, familiar to all: coffee, tea and chocolate, which are rich in caffeine, theobromine and related alkaloids, are regularly used as a short-term restorative to keep students and night owls awake. They are, however, superficial remedies offering no real long-term benefits when it comes to improving energy levels and strengthening the nervous system. A better alternative is rosemary, which contains a stimulant called borneal. Taken as an infusion it can effectively ease short-term fatigue problems while a few drops of rosemary oil added to bath water is a stimulating and refreshing way to start the day. Guarana, a popular over-the-counter restorative, is another: here the action is largely dependent on caffeine-like stimulants, although in this case the guaranine alkaloid is much slower to metabolise so has a gentler, more sustained effect.

Longer-term energy tonics are often a better option: Korean ginseng is now well established in the West as a tonic remedy. In traditional Chinese medicine, Korean ginseng tends to be regarded as boosting the masculine (*yang*) energies and, while it can obviously be taken by women without ill-effects, other tonics may often be preferable. *Dang Shen*, American ginseng and Siberian ginseng are all regarded as less aggressive and rather more feminine (*yin*) in character. In China *Huang Qi* (milk vetch) is often preferred for younger people with Korean ginseng reserved for the over-forties. Becoming more popular in the West are Ayurvedic tonic remedies, such as *ashwagandha* and *shatavari* which can also be useful to counter excessive tiredness.

If a stressful time is looming – such as exams or a heavy work period – then it is worth taking tonic herbs before the event to provide an energy boost, rather than depending on short-term stimulants once the stresses mount. Herbs such as Siberian ginseng and golden root are particularly useful for helping the body cope more efficiently with stress and improving performance. Siberian ginseng was widely used in the 1960s and '70s by Soviet athletes and long-distance lorry-drivers to increase stamina. Golden root – also sold as rhodiola – has been used medicinally since the days of Dioscorides, and has always been especially popular in the folk medicine of Russia and Scandinavia where it grows abundantly. Today, golden root is increasingly popular as an over-the-counter remedy used for a wide range of nervous and stress-related disorders including chronic fatigue syndrome, post-traumatic stress disorder and attention deficit problems in children.

While all these herbal remedies have a place and can be very effective, they are not a total solution. If fatigue is due to overwork or a dysfunctional lifestyle then the problem will only be solved if that, too, changes.

Chinese medicine reserves the powerful tonic remedies for obvious energy-deficiency syndromes rather than using them as a convenient top-up. Their use is almost always combined with exercise therapies such as *Qigong* or *t'ai-chi.* In Ayurveda – which translates as the 'science of life' – treatment for energy weakness will similarly always involve meditation, dietary changes, *hatha yoga* or gem therapy. Both approaches also emphasise the spiritual and emotional sides of life, blaming exhaustion not only on physical imbalance but on a lack of spirituality in our lives.

Headaches

Headaches are generally symptoms of some underlying disorder rather than illnesses in their own right. Causes are numerous and the location and character of the pain is often an indication of what that underlying problem might be. Those centred behind the eyes, for example, can suggest a digestive disturbance, while pain and sensitivity around the eyes or above the nose can be caused by a sinus problem. Headaches that seem to start at the back of the neck and creep forward are generally tension related.

These headaches usually start with a tightening of the muscles at the back of the neck and then creep forward until the whole head is painful. They can often be associated with physical muscle strain in the shoulders and neck from sitting or working awkwardly, hunched over a desk or computer keyboard but, just as commonly, the physical tightening is linked to mental stress.

For some people, tension headaches are extremely common at stressful times; others may find that stress highlights a different area of weakness with stomach upsets or urinary problems. Relaxing herbs such as vervain, wood betony, skullcap, chamomile, valerian, lavender and St John's wort can ease symptoms, while Siberian ginseng can improve one's stress tolerance and thus reduce the risk of headaches in the first place. Symptomatic treatment can involve massage using soothing oils, like lavender, across the neck or temples.

Migraine is an especially common problem and is typically preceded by visual disturbances: jagged lights at the edge of the visual field or a sense that there is a strange out-of-focus area in what one sees. Identifying the cause is again important: this may be food intolerance or stress-related. Red wine, chocolate, pork, citrus fruits, coffee and cheese are all common culprits.

Many sufferers find that chewing feverfew leaves can help prevent attacks, although this herb can cause ulceration of the mucous membranes (usually in the form of mouth ulcers) in sensitive individuals and it should not be taken if this side-effect develops. Lavender oil massaged into the temples can sometimes help prevent an attack developing, while valerian and wood betony taken internally can also be useful.

In Chinese medicine headaches are defined either in terms of inner organ imbalance or external factors. Practitioners look for associated symptoms which pinpoint the problem: dizziness and ringing in the ears, for example, may suggest a kidney deficiency syndrome. The kidneys are also associated with the emotion 'fear' which may also play a part in anxiety problems.

Headaches linked to anxiety are seen in Ayurveda are commonly related to the *vata* (wind) humour and may also be associated with dry skin, irregular diet, excessive activity and constipation. Sedating herbs and purgatives are likely to be used. *Pitta* (bile) headaches are more likely to be associated with irritability and anger and may be treated with liver herbs such as *gotu kola*. Anxiety and stress is also believed to damage the essential vigour or energy of the body so supporting tonic herbs, such as *shatavari* or *ashwagandha,* will often be added where headaches are a persistent problem.

Persistent or sudden unusually severe headaches lasting for three days or more should be referred to a medical practitioner.

Heart and blood pressure problems

While orthodox western medicine regards the heart as little more than a mechanical pump (as discussed in Chapter 1) traditional approaches to healing imbue it with a range of emotional and spiritual attributes. For the Chinese it controls the life process; co-ordinates the activities of all the other organs; manages mental activities and consciousness; and is the storehouse of *Shen* – a sense of appropriateness and right behaviour. In Ayurveda it is the dwelling place of the *atman* – the divine self or spirit of immortal life.

Significantly several recent studies (O'Connor *et al.*, 2000; Gorman and Sloan, 2000; Krishnan, 2000; Pitzalis *et al.*, 2001; Abramson *et al.*, 2001) have demonstrated a link between depressive illness and heart disease. These studies have shown that the risk of heart attack among older, depressed patients is twice that of those with a more positive outlook. The depressed group was also more likely to suffer from strokes, while depressed patients were less likely to make a good recovery from either a heart attack or a stroke. Anxiety was less closely linked with heart problems but people suffering from high levels of daily mental stress were also found to be more at risk of heart and cardiovascular disorders.

Personality, too, plays a part and it has long been established that the more relaxed and laid back about life we are (type B personality), then the less likely we are to suffer from heart disorders. The 'type A' individuals with a more aggressive, ambitious and time-pressured approach to daily life, constantly striving to meet self-imposed deadlines, are far more likely candidates for heart problems.

Prolonged high blood pressure (hypertension) can be a precursor to more severe health problems, putting excessive strain on heart muscles and damaging the cardiovascular system. In around 90 per cent of cases there is no clear cause for the problem; in a minority of instances kidney disease, glandular problems or pregnancy may be the trigger. Contributory risk factors can include obesity, a sedentary lifestyle, high salt intake, smoking and prolonged excessive stress.

In the past cholesterol has often been blamed for the problem. Cholesterol is a complex fatty substance which is essential for physical health. The average body contains about 150g of cholesterol and it plays an important role in maintaining membrane fluidity, as well as providing the raw material for manufacturing many hormones and bile acids. This useful substance has, however, been associated with fatty deposits developing in blood vessels, which in turn leads to narrowing of the arteries and increased blood pressure. Cholesterol is a naturally occurring substance and some studies have suggested that artificially reducing it with drugs just encourages the body to produce yet more. The debate continues, but the anti-animal-fat messages which were so common a few years ago are being modified and there is a growing realisation that a little cholesterol in the diet may be no bad thing.

Numerous herbs can, however, help to control the levels of surplus cholesterol in the blood and encourage its excretion; much research has focused on garlic, which has been proven to help reduce the risk of a further heart attack in those already suffering problems with damage blood vessels and hardened arteries. Daily doses of 1–4 cloves per person have been suggested as ideal – which is no more than one could easily use in cooking. German trials suggest that 2g a day of powdered garlic is sufficient to achieve notable therapeutic effects.

Other foodstuffs which have been shown to have a similar cholesterol-modifying action include chickpeas, kidney beans, navy beans (the sort that go into cans of baked beans), lentils, soya beans and alfalfa sprouts. Herbs showing the same properties include nutmeg, sage, linden, thyme, garlic, liquorice and ginseng.

Isolated blood pressure readings really mean very little: several consistently high ones are needed before applying the label 'hypertension' and mild cases can often be controlled by simple dietary measures. Coffee, for example, contains caffeine which stimulates the heart to beat faster, pumping blood through the vessels and kidneys more energetically. The result – even in healthy people – can be an abnormally fast pulse, irregular heart beat, raised blood pressure and increased desire to urinate. Often simply cutting down on coffee – along with tea and chocolate, which contain similar chemicals – is all that is needed.

While the precise cause of raised blood pressure may be unknown, it makes sense for sufferers to attempt at least to combat known causal factors: losing weight, stopping smoking, taking more exercise and learning to relax more effectively are sensible stratagems for sufferers.

Herbs can be used to combat specific symptoms – diuretics or cardiovascular relaxants to reduce blood pressure on a simple mechanical basis, for example, or heart tonics and restoratives to help strengthen a possibly weakened system. Among the more commonly used are hawthorn, which is a good heart tonic and also generally helps to lower raised blood pressure; garlic, cramp bark, yarrow, and dandelion leaves. Suitably relaxing herbs to combat any contributory stress and anxiety include valerian. linden, vervain, and passion flower. Motherwort can be especially helpful if palpitations are a problem.

A typical infusion for raised blood pressure is:

2 parts hawthorn flowers
2 parts lime flowers
1 part dandelion leaf

1 part yarrow
1 part vervain or passion flower

One teaspoon of the mixture infused with a cup of boiling water to be taken two or three times a day.

Insomnia

The amount of sleep we each need varies considerably and sometimes we require rather more sleep than at others. Dark mornings in the winter encourage us to stay in bed for longer while bright sunshine before five a.m. on a midsummer day encourages us to leap up, feeling refreshed and energised. Lying awake and relaxed all night is not necessarily a problem and sleeplessness only becomes an issue when sufferers feel tired and unable to concentrate during the day or when it becomes a worry in itself.

Our society tends to be rather preoccupied about the amount and quality of sleep we each achieve and, as alternative therapy practitioners know only too well, sleep problems rank high in a 'top ten' of presenting ailments.

There are many causes for disturbed sleep patterns: heavy meals late at night can lead to disturbed digestion; painful joints and muscles or irritating coughs will keep most people awake; while catnapping during the day simply fills up the sleep quota and there is no need for further rest. Drinking beverages containing caffeine or caffeine-like compounds – such as coffee, commercial 'cola' drinks, chocolate and tea – late at night can also be a problem for some people and it is always a good idea to stop any stimulating mental activity at least an hour before bed. Rudolf Steiner, originator of many anthroposophical remedies, maintained that one should never undertake mental work after eight p.m. at night as this interfered too much with daily rhythms.

And then there is worry: reliving arguments with loved ones, rehearsing the next day's key meeting or interview, and so on – it all so easily culminates in a restless night. Most of us can exist on far less sleep than we believe is essential. There is an old Chinese saying to the effect that a woman needs six hours sleep, a man seven and only a fool needs eight. Few would wholeheartedly agree with such beliefs, but it is certainly true that the amount of sleep we each need varies and that at some times we need rather more sleep than others.

Sleep disorders are generally divided into two broad groups: problems getting to sleep or waking after a few hours and finding it difficult to get back to sleep again. Common causes in the first category include stress, anxiety, stimulants (such as caffeine), pain and emotional problems. In the second more complex health issues can be involved such as breathing difficulties, restless leg syndrome (involuntary twitching of the leg muscles), depression, pain, low blood sugar or snoring.

In Chinese theory *Qi* (our vital energy) moves around the body during the space of twenty-four hours, so waking at a particular time may be associated with an imbalance in that particular organ and this would guide treatment (see Table 7).

Table 7: The daily Qi timetable

Time	Meridians
3–5a.m.	Lung
5–7a.m.	Large Intestine
7–9a.m.	Stomach
9–11a.m.	Spleen
11a.m.–1p.m.	Heart
1–3p.m.	Small Intestine
3p.m.–5p.m.	Urinary Bladder
5p.m.–7p.m.	Kidney
7–9p.m.	Pericardium
9–11p.m.	Triple Burner*
11p.m.–1a.m.	Gall Bladder
1–3a.m.	Liver

* A Chinese organ concept roughly equivalent to the upper, central and lower abdomen and covering digestive function.

Insomnia is commonly associated with tension, worries and a failure to relax before bedtime – an aspect of anxiety that can respond well to sedating herbs such as chamomile, lemon balm, skullcap, Californian poppy, vervain, lavender or St John's wort. Insomnia can also be due to over-excitement, manic or behaviour or hysteria. Particularly effective here can be cowslip petals although you do need rather a lot of them to make a suitable cup of tea.

Numerous over-the-counter herbal products are available for insomnia. Many contain valerian, hops, wild lettuce or passion flower, with Californian poppy included in more recently developed brands. Until recently kava, too, was recommended for insomnia, although recent restrictions on its sale have rather limited its availability.

Most herbal remedies need to be taken up to an hour before bedtime. An exception is kava which can take time to develop its soporific action, so is best taken earlier in the evening so that a period of calm, relaxation with enhanced mental awareness can be followed by natural sleep.

Herbal remedies for insomniacs can be combined in many different ways to provide pleasant tasting teas. One effective combination uses:

1 part skullcap or wood betony
1 part lavender flowers
2 parts passion flower
2 parts Californian poppy

Shake the herbs together well in a small jar and then infuse one to two teaspoons in a cup of boiling water for five minutes, strain into a clean cup before drinking about thirty minutes before bedtime.

As always with herbal medicine, it is far better to identify and treat the cause of a problem rather than simply tackle the symptoms, so if inability to relax or over-anxiety is the root cause of insomnia, meditation classes or a review of lifestyle concerns might provide the solution.

Unlike orthodox treatments herbal insomnia remedies are non-addictive, although some people find that their potency is reduced if they take it regularly, so it can be worthwhile changing the mix from time to time in long-term use.

Seasonal affective disorder (SAD)

In temperate climates, seasonal affective disorder (SAD), most commonly occurs as recurrent winter depression. As the days grow shorter and sunshine less common, sufferers become more and more depressed with lethargy, sleep disturbances, irritability, poor concentration, reduced libido and social withdrawal.

The syndrome has been linked to melatonin production. This is one of the body's hormones which is produced according to the presence or absence of daylight. In hibernating animals, melatonin production increases as the days get shorter and this acts to slow down the body's physiology, encourage weight increase and finally sends many hundreds of animal species into a long sleep to avoid the worst of the winter weather.

Researchers have found that exposing SAD sufferers to higher levels of light can change their melatonin production pattern and help reduce the familiar symptoms of winter depression. Typical working environments have light levels of around 500 lux, a sunny English garden is around 2,000 lux and a Mediterranean beach around 5,000 lux (van Straten, 1993) so a major increase in ambient light levels is needed by sufferers. Numerous light boxes and daylight simulation lamps are now available for home use. These are most effective when used to simulate morning light although latest studies suggest that as long as the light simulation is given at around dawn (Eagles, 2001) it need not be quite so luminously bright as therapy at other times of the day.

Herbs used for depression can be just as effective for SAD with St John's wort (Wheatley, 1999) proving particularly useful in trials – although as one might expect the best results were obtained from a mixture of St John's wort, providing symptomatic relief, and regular treatment from a bright light source, to treat the underlying cause. Lemon balm, wood betony, wild oats, basil and vervain can also be helpful.

As well as anti-depressants, using gentle stimulants to combat feelings of lethargy and apathy is also important. Guarana is preferred by some as a more gentle caffeine-like stimulant, while other herbalists suggest kola nuts, *gotu kola,* rosemary, or Korean ginseng; *Dang Shen* or American ginseng may be preferable for some as they are rather more gentle than the Korean variety.

Spiritual problems

As we have seen, traditional theories of medicine – still practised in traditional Chinese and Ayurvedic medicine – made little divide between physical, emotional and spiritual aspects of our being. Good health was believed to depend not only on physical well-being but on mental balance and spiritual harmony. These beliefs go back to a time before our western 'Age of Enlightenment'.

Today, talk of spiritual matters has become rather unfashionable: the main emphases in our society are on possessions, work and socialising. Support for conventional religion has dwindled, for a minority off-beat New Age cults become ever more bizarre, while the vast majority of us have been far too busy 'getting and spending' to devote much time to this side of our nature. Focusing on the old-fashioned 'virtues' of compassion, generosity, charity and kindness might just be rather better for our over-all well-being than too much greed, envy, self-interest or acquisitiveness.

Until well into the seventeenth century faith and religious belief were inextricably tangled with 'science' and medicine. Illness was as much due to spiritual transgression as invading micro-organisms and a priest/shaman was essential to effect any cure. Old herbals frequently combine prayers with a list of herbal remedies and in earlier ages the healing powers of plants would have been enhanced by gathering them at sacred times or praying to relevant deities. In traditional societies even today the shaman continues to combine incantations, herbs and trance states in an attempt to visit the spirit world and persuade whatever is troubling the patient to depart.

The Cherokee in North America, for example, believed that rheumatism was caused by the revengeful spirits of slain deer so the shaman had to invoke the wolf and dog spirits, powerful enemies of the deer, to help him to cure the ailment. Hallucinogenic herbs were used to help the shaman enter this spirit world: peyote taken by Mexican shaman or fly agaric used by Siberian healers, for example.

Eastern healing traditions, too, do not separate the spiritual from the physical. In Tibetan medicine, for example, there is strong emphasis on the effects of past lives and deeds – *karma* – on one's health in the present. The exact time when symptoms appeared would be matched to astrological charts to identify the cause of the problem. Treatment was also multi-dimensional: herbal medicines prepared with great ritual with the physician using meditation and special mantras to energise the remedy and increase its efficacy, while patients, too, would be expected to combine spiritual exercises with their patent nostrums.

Ayurvedic theory – like traditional Chinese medicine – has its roots in early philosophy dating back at least 2,500 years and over the centuries has developed a complex integrated model in which the physical is inseparable from both spiritual issues and the wider world around us. The theory is based on a triad of cosmic forces: *prana*, the breath of life; *agni,* the spirit of light or fire, and *soma*, a manifestation of harmony, cohesiveness and love. This creation as a continuous interchange between the two basic principles: *praktri* – unconscious nature or energy and *purusha* – consciousness or matter.

Purusha is then further divided into the three essential qualities or *gunas*: *sattva* which can be translated as cognition or clarity, *rajas* – action, and *tamas* – desire or substance. These three qualities give rise to the three psychic forces: *buddhi* – intellect;

ahamkara – ego; and *manas* – mind or spirit. For good health. balance is also needed among the three *gunas. Sattva* is regarded as purity and enlightenment while *rajas* and *tamas* can be seen as representing the darker side of nature – respectively distraction and dullness. Spiritual health is maintained by learning to control *rajas* and *tamas* while developing the calm, clarity of *sattva*.

Just as the herbs used in Ayurveda and TCM have physical properties which can be defined in acceptable scientific language – for example as anti-inflammatories, anti-depressants, expectorants or relaxants – so do they also have less tangible qualities.

Ayurvedic tonic herbs are classified as:

- nutritive to strengthen the body
- aphrodisiac to reinvigorate the sexual organs and inner energies, or
- rejuvenative to help creativity and awareness.

Nutritive tonics *(bruhana karma)* tend to be sweet in taste.

Aphrodisiac remedies are known as *vajikarana*, from *'vaji'* a stallion – renowned in Indian tradition for its sexual activity. They are believed not only to bring the energy and vitality of a horse, but to focus on reproductive energy and help energise all the body's tissues. By increasing sexual energy the *vajikarana* help to create new life in conception as well as help to renew our own lives.

The rejuvenative remedies (*rasayana karma*) are among the most important in Ayurveda and are sometimes called longevity tonics. *Rasayana* tonics are also described as rejuvenating remedies to renew mind, body and spirit and combat ageing and decay. Like the nutritive tonics, many are sweet to taste but there are also pungent, hot spicy remedies that are particularly appropriate for some conditions. In Ayurvedic theory plants possess a substance called *soma* which is an almost magical nectar to renew the whole being and *rasayanas* are believed to provide plenty of this vital energy-giving substance to increase understanding and awareness.

Among the more important *rasayanas* are: *ashwagandha*, guggul, aloe vera, *gotu kola*, saffron, *shatavari*, *jatamansi*, and *jati* (jasmine). Western herbs, too, have these subtle spiritual attributes – although much traditional knowledge is now deeply buried in ancient manuscripts.

CHAPTER 4

Helpful herbs

> All nature is like one single apothercary's shop, covered only with the roof of heaven; and only One Being works the pestle as far as the world extends. But man has such a shop only in part, not wholly; he possesses something, not everything. For nature's apothecary's shop is greater than man's.
>
> Paracelsus (1493–1541)

Calming herbs and relaxation techniques can be used to combat the body's need for that stressful adrenaline rush, so reducing the likelihood of springing into 'panic mode' without due cause. The herbal repertoire includes a great many nervines which soothe and restore the nervous system to encourage greater relaxation and restful sleep, as well as others to help raise the stress threshold so that the damaging 'flight or fight' response is reserved for real crises.

There are also many stimulating remedies to help strengthen what Victorian herbalists described as 'the vital force' and boost energy levels to combat exhaustion and over-work.

Many herbs can also influence our emotional and spiritual well-being. Plants like *reishi* mushroom and basil have been used for centuries in Eastern cultures to promote inner calm and compassion. Others, such as kava, have been widely misused in western society because of their psychoactive properties.

Mostly calming

Many western herbs are defined as sedative, relaxing or tranquillising. Their action is often complex and not fully understood. Passion flower, for example, is known to prolong sleep times and reduce locomotor activity but the constituent responsible for the action has yet to be identified. Chamomile, similarly, is found by many to be calming and relaxing yet research studies have generally only been able to identify anti-inflammatory, anti-bacterial, anti-spasmodic and immune stimulating activity.

Eastern remedies often adopt a rather more spiritual emphasis focusing on herbs which can encourage feelings of compassion and love – the *sattvic* remedies of Ayurveda, for example – rather than simply focusing on demonstrable physical relaxation.

The remedies listed in this section are often suitable for anxiety, nervous tension, and such stress-related problems as an inability to relax and unwind or emotional upsets.

MUGWORT

Botanical name: Artemisia vulgaris

Parts used: leaves

How to use: infusions – 15g of dried herb to 500ml boiling water taken in three equal doses; tincture – up to 10 drops, three times a day

To the Anglo-Saxons mugwort was one of the 'nine sacred herbs' given to the world by the god Woden and described in the ninth century poem, *Lacnunga* as:

> . . .eldest of worts, thou has might for three and against thirty; for venom availest, for flying vile things; mighty gainst loathed ones that through the land rove. . .

The herb was believed to be a potent totem against evil and surviving Anglo-Saxon herbals suggest hanging a root of it over the doorway of a house to prevent both it and its inhabitants coming to any harm; sprigs were regularly worn to avert the evil eye. Even today sprigs of mugwort are still worn on the opening day of the Isle of Man parliament – the UK's oldest civic gathering. The herb was believed to protect buildings from lightning strikes. The name mugwort reputedly derives from the Saxon '*mugga wort*' or midge plant as it will also effectively repel insects.

More practically, the Romans are believed to have planted mugwort alongside their roads so that they could line their sandals with the herb on a long journey to prevent aching feet. Today, it is still very commonly found growing alongside old roads. The Roman naturalist, Pliny, recommends carrying sprigs of mugwort on a journey to prevent both tiredness and attacks by wild animals. Traditionally mugwort pillows were used to encourage prophetic dreams: a mixture of bay, mugwort and rosemary was considered especially effective for the purpose.

Mugwort is a bitter digestive stimulant, still occasionally used in cooking. It can be added to stuffings for fatty meats like goose. The herb is a mild sedative and also effects the gynaecological system so is mainly used for menstrual problems associated with nervous tension; as a calming remedy for emotional upsets it is especially valuable at the menopause. It combines well with sage in teas for menopausal problems or can help normalise irregular menstrual activity.

In the East, a local variety of mugwort leaf (*A. vulgaris*, var. *indicus* known as *Ai Ye* in Mandarin) is used as *moxa* – sticks or cones of dried herb that are burned at the end of acupuncture needles (moxibustion) for 'cold' conditions like arthritis. In Ayurvedic medicine mugwort is used to help the brow and throat *chakras* to improve concentration and creativity and to help strengthen our inner resources.

Caution: avoid mugwort in pregnancy; do not use in epilepsy.

CALIFORNIAN POPPY

Botanical name: Eschscholzia californica

Parts used: aerial parts

How to use: capsules – 2–3 at night; infusion – 1–3 teaspoons per cup of boiling water at night for insomnia for adults or ½–1 teaspoon for children or 25g to 500ml boiling water in three equal doses for general use

Californian poppies are a popular and easy-to-grow garden plant with cheerful bright orange flowers. A member of the poppy family, the herb shares the sedative and hypnotic effects of its more powerful cousin – the opium poppy. However, its mix of alkaloids is rather different and instead of the potent morphine and codeine type alkaloids of opium, it contains rather gentler isoquinoline alkaloids such as protopine, cryptopine and chelidine. Californian poppy is thus a mild sedative and sleep-inducing herb, suitable even for restless children; it is also diaphoretic (encourages sweating) so can be a useful cooling sedative in feverish illnesses. In North America it has the country name of 'nightcap'.

The plant is also effective at relieving pain and was used by Native Americans as an internal remedy for colic and gastric pains. It is a mild diuretic and can be useful in urinary tract disorders such as cystitis.

However, it is poorly researched and one is again dependent on anecdotal reports suggesting that it can be helpful in various nervous conditions, including bedwetting in children, bladder and urinary disorders and various painful conditions. Californian poppy is combined with oat extract in the German proprietary remedy, Requiesan, marketed as a calming sedative (Weiss, 1988)

California poppy is extremely easy to grow in the garden; seeds are readily available from garden centres and, although an annual, once established the plant will continue to self-seed to establish a permanent clump than needs very little attention. It is easy to gather the whole herb during the flowering season, dry in small bunches and store for use as a night-time tea to combat insomnia or anxiety.

Some remedies include the root as well – this is quite shallow and comes up easily when pulling handfuls of the plant. Be sure to leave some in the garden, however, to seed for the following year.

HOPS

Botanical name: Humulus lupulus

Part used: strobiles (flowers from female plants)

How to use: tincture – up to 2ml/40 drops, three times a day; infusion – 15g to 500ml of boiling water taken in three equal doses

Although we associate hops with traditional English beer, the plant is a comparative newcomer, introduced from Germany in the sixteenth century. Enthusing about the hop plant's many virtues, John Gerard, writing in 1597, urges that 'beer' be considered a 'phisicall drink to keep the body in health [rather] than an ordinary drinke for the quenching of our thirst', while a few years earlier (1562) William Turner in his *New Herball* was amazed that, given the herb's numerous properties, physicians did not 'use it more in medicine'. Just as in brewing, the female flowers or strobiles are used medicinally.

Hops have been used for many years as a sedative but why they act in this way is not fully understood despite extensive investigations into the plant's active constituents. Among the various chemicals hops contain are a group known as phloroglucinol derivatives which are largely in the form of ketones. These include humulone and lupulone which gradually degrade during storage so that the properties of hops can vary depending on the age of the dried herb. There is also a complex volatile oil which also changes over time so that old hops are found to contain significant amounts of a chemical called 2–methyl–3-buten–2-ol, for example, while only minute traces of this are found in the fresh plant.

The chemical mix in fresh hops is generally considered better for insomnia: pillows filled with the strobiles are a popular folk remedy for sleeplessness but they really only work with fresh herbs – as the strobiles dry and the chemicals change the pillow becomes less effective. Hops in such pillows need to be changed every few months to ensure continuing activity.

Older dried hops tend to be more restorative for the nervous system so can be better for exhaustion and stress. The 2–methyl–3-buten–2-ol which develops as the herb ages has been shown to have a depressant effect on the central nervous system and this chemical is known to be similar in form to the sedative drug methylpentynol (Wohlfart *et al.*, 1983).

Hops contain chemicals which are very similar to the female sex hormone oestrogen so it tends to reduce the male libido – an action which may be familiar to beer drinkers: excessive consumption can also lead to an increase in external female sexual characteristics. In the past women hop pickers often experienced menstrual irregularities and early periods while working in the hop fields and inhaling the herb's potent aromatic oils. Hops can also relieve abdominal cramps and are bitter tasting to stimulate the digestion.

Hops are generally regarded as quite safe and non-toxic with no reported side-effects. They are officially recommended across Europe for sleep disorders and for restlessness and excitability associated with anxiety.

Caution: hops are strongly sedating, and are best avoided by those liable to nervous depression.

JASMINE

Botanical name: Jasminium spp.

Parts used: flowers, essential oil

How to use: essential oil – use 1–2 drops to 5ml of wheatgerm oil in massage rubs

Common jasmine *(J. officinale)* is a highly aromatic climbing plant, introduced into Europe in the sixteenth century and popular today as both an aromatic house plant and a vigorous climber in warmer, sheltered areas. The plant rapidly gained popularity with the French perfumiers who developed a technique for extracting the richly scented oil using *enfleurage.* This method involves layering the flowers (which must be picked in the evening when the scent is strongest) with wax between glass sheets. The stack of wax and glass is left for several days until the aromatic oils in the jasmine have been absorbed into the wax. The wax is then stripped from the glass, melted and the oil separated from the waxy layer.

Producing jasmine oil is highly expensive and labour intensive process and not surprisingly the result is often adulterated with synthetic chemicals; only the very best grades should be used medicinally. In aromatherapy it is included in massage rubs for period pain, anxiety, insomnia, and depression, impotence and frigidity, and for abdominal massage during childbirth to encourage parturition and ease labour pains. It is also added to chest rubs for coughs and breathing difficulties.

Jasmine contains a number of alkaloids (including jasminine) while the essential oil is rich in benzyl alcohol, linalool, and linyl acetate; the herb also contains salicylic acid, which is similar to the chemical used in aspirin, so is analgesic and cooling to reduce fevers.

A close relative, royal jasmine or *jati (J. grandiflorum)* is an important Ayurvedic tonic and cleansing remedy. *Jati* is regarded as a *sattvic* tonic – encouraging principles of light, perception and harmony. The flowers are regarded as mildly aphrodisiac for women and also cleansing for the uterus, while their *sattvic* nature also emphasises love and compassion. *Jati* is used in infections to reduce fevers and strengthen the immune system. The herb can be combined with lemon balm or skullcap to make a calming tea ideal at the end of a stressful day.

Jasmine tea, popular in China, is scented with yet another variety – *J. sambac* or Arabian jasmine which originates in the Persian Gulf. Arabian jasmine has been used for scenting Chinese teas since at least AD300. Traditionally the flowers, known as *Mo Li,* would simply be left next to heat-dried green tea for several hours to absorb the scent. Modern commercial producers generally just mix the petals with the tea instead. According to Li Shi Zhen (1578) jasmine tea is soothing and warming and will help relieve diarrhoea. It is more popular in Northern China than in the South.

If available, *jati* is the preferable internal remedy: the tea is soothing and relaxing to combat stress and anxiety while helping to increase mental clarity and awareness. Jasmine oil, as a massage, is almost as good although without the comfort factor of a nice relaxed cup of tea – try drinking Chinese jasmine tea after massaging with jasmine oil to achieve the double effect.

WILD LETTUCE

Botanical name: Lactuca virosa

Parts used: aerial parts, dried juice

How to use: fresh lettuce – eat at the start of a meal as a digestive stimulant; decoction – use 75g to 750ml of water in a decoction, simmered for thirty minutes and taken in wineglass doses after meals as a digestive remedy and mild sedative or externally as a lotion for acne; pulp a whole fresh lettuce in a food processor and take in 10ml doses for period pains; wild lettuce tincture – up to 5ml at night for insomnia or 1–2ml, three times daily for nervous tension

As Peter Rabbit memorably discovered, eating plenty of lettuce – especially if it has bolted and is going to seed – can make you very sleepy. Wild lettuce *(L. virosa)* is used in herbal medicine, as a potent sedative and painkiller, but cultivated varieties have a long history of healing uses as well.

The cos lettuce was grown in Ancient Egypt and held sacred to Min, the god of fertility – probably because its milky juice was thought to resemble semen. This lettuce latex was used by the Assyrians as a cough mixture and until the 1930s similar dried juice extracted from the wild lettuce was sold in British pharmacies as 'lettuce opium' and applied in much the same way as the rather more potent drug. Despite Egyptian preoccupations, lettuce latex is generally regarded as an anaphrodisiac and the herb was known as 'the eunuch's plant' in ancient Greece.

Lettuce latex was obtained by repeatedly slicing off the top of the growing lettuce stem and then collecting the exuded white sap which was then dried. This latex contains chemicals known as sesquiterpene lactones including lactucopicrin and lactucerin.

There is are also coumarins, sugars (mannitol) and flavonoids including apigenin and quercitin. Reports around 1900 suggested that fresh lettuce also contained hyoscyamine, which is a very potent alkaloid found in members of the Solanaceae family including deadly nightshade, but this has never been detected in the dried extract. Some studies also detected low levels of morphine in lettuce but the quantity is too minute to have any therapeutic action.

Lettuce opium is rarely produced commercially these days and modern herbalists tend to use the dried leaf or tinctures made from the whole aerial part of the plant. It tends to be at its most potent before flowering – long after the plant would have been collected for use in salads. The dried leaves were also once incorporated into herbal smoking mixtures which were used as calming remedies for asthma and bronchitis, although these are less common nowadays.

Like other long-established herbal remedies, there has been little research into the sedative properties of lettuce (Bradley, 1992; Newall *et al.*, 1996); one study in the 1980s appears to have demonstrated a sedative effect on toads of extracts from cultivated lettuce samples, but there have been no significant clinical trials to confirm the herb's traditional uses.

The cultivated lettuce is milder in action than its wild cousin, but can also be used as a cleansing, mildly laxative and digestive stimulant. Serving lettuce as a first course can help stimulate the digestion for heavier instalments of the meal. As a cleansing remedy lettuce – both wild and cultivated – can be helpful for various arthritic problems and constipation. It has also been used for period pains, liver congestion and a variety of nervous disorders and over-excitement (including hyperactivity in children).

Herbalists tend to use wild lettuce extracts for insomnia and for persistent, irritant coughs. The plant can also be helpful for rheumatic pains and especially useful for soothing irritable and restless children.

Caution: skin rashes have been reported among agricultural workers cutting large quantities of cultivated lettuce but there are no documented reports of side-effects for wild lettuce.

LAVENDER

Botanical name: Lavandula angustifolia

Parts used: flowers, essential oil

How to use: tincture – up to 4ml/80 drops, three times a day; infusion – 25g dried flowers to 500ml boiling water, three times daily; essential oil – add 5–10 drops to 5ml of almond oil and use for massage

The name lavender comes from the Latin *lavare*, to wash, and the herb has been used to scent baths and toiletries since Roman times. Lavender is useful for digestive upsets, nervous tension, insomnia, migraines and headaches. It is a mild painkiller and anti-depressant that will also relieve muscular spasms and cramps. The flowers can be made into a pleasant tasting tea that can be taken at night for sleeplessness or during the day for headaches and nervous tension. Pillows containing lavender flowers, especially when combined with chamomile flowers, are a traditional remedy for easing a troubled mind, while a sleep pillow with lavender and orange blossoms is more likely to improve mental clarity.

Dioscorides, writing in the second century AD, recommended lavender for 'griefs in the thorax', although the plant used by the Greeks was probably *L. stoechas,* generally known today as French lavender and rather less hardy than the familiar English variety. In Arabic medicine this tradition of using lavender for chest problems has continued and it is still used in the Middle East as a cough remedy. Herbalists usually describe lavender as 'cooling', suggesting that it is best suited to ease those sorts of headaches that are soothed by cold packs rather than the sort of pain that is comforted by a warm compress.

Most of lavender's active constituents are packed into the essential oil which is collected by steam-distillation of the flowers. One of the most abundant chemicals is linalyl acetate while others include linalool, lavandulyl acetate, borneol and camphor. There are also coumarins, which among other properties, reduce the stickiness of the blood, and flavonoids which can affect the blood vessels.

Although herbalists still recommend infusions or tinctures of lavender flowers for insomnia and anxiety, the herb is best known in aromatherapy where the essential oil is used in massage treatments for muscular aches, pains and headaches, for inflammations and catarrh, and to ease digestive problems. Studies suggest that just sniffing the oil can have a sedative effect (Buchbauer *et al.*, 1991).

A few drops of lavender oil can also be added to creams for eczema or diluted in water to make a soothing lotion for sunburn and minor scalds. Added to bath water, lavender oil is relaxing and soothing for nervous tensions and insomnia; in massage oils it can be helpful for muscular aches and pains, strains and some rheumatic problems. As often happens, few of these uses have been investigated by researchers so many are dismissed as unsubstantiated folklore.

Traditionally lavender has also been used as a heart tonic – calming what Nicholas Culpeper described in 1653 as 'tremblings and passions of the heart'; a description which aromatherapist Robert Tisserand (1977) says describes 'the kind of mental state in which lavender is indicated'. This could include feelings of panic, irritability, indecision, hysteria and trembling which can be associated with the more extreme manifestations of 'anxiety'.

Lavender works well in combinations: the flower tea is a

sedating, calming mixture to encourage relaxation and rest with the concurrent use of the essential oil externally in massage, as a muscle relaxant and relief for spasmodic pains. The plant is generally regarded as very safe with no real concerns over toxicity, although, like all essential oils, it is best avoided in pregnancy.

MOTHERWORT

Botanical name: Leonurus cardiaca

Parts used: leaves, seeds

How to use: infusion – 25g of dried herb to 500ml boiling water taken in three equal doses; tincture – up to 5ml, three times daily

Motherwort is used today mainly as a heart tonic and sedative. It reputedly takes its common name from a traditional use to calm anxiety in mothers during childbirth or as John Gerard put it in 1597: 'for them that are in hard travell with childe'. The *Leonurus* part of the botanical name is from a Greek word meaning lion's tail and describes the shaggy shape of the leaves, while *cardiaca* reminds us that this has been an important heart herb since Roman times. The plant belongs to the mint family, and like others in the group, motherwort is a rather drab plant with tiny pink flowers clustered at the axil where the leaves join the main stem.

Motherwort can help to steady erratic heart beats and ease palpitations while more recent research also suggests that it can help prevent thromboses (blood clots) and reduce the stickiness of the blood which can lead to circulatory disorders (McCaleb, 1990). A study involving 105 patients using the herb as a blood thinner found significant reduction in associated symptoms such as numbness, insomnia and headaches.

As a mild sedative, the herb is helpful for treating menopausal upsets and associated palpitations: it works well in infusions in combination with sage or mugwort to relieve a wide spectrum of menopausal discomforts. As its traditional use in childbirth suggests it is also a uterine stimulant so can be helpful for some types of menstrual disorders and period pains.

Motherwort is a useful sedative, especially in emotional upsets associated with the menopause and is also worth adding to mixtures for severe anxiety to ease the palpitations common in panic attacks.

A related species, *L. heterophyllus*, is used in China mainly for menstrual problems. The leaves are known as *Yi Mu Cao* and are also used for some sorts of eczema while the seeds are called *Chong Wei Zi* and are included in remedies for eye problems such as conjunctivitis.

Caution: avoid high doses in pregnancy.

CHAMOMILE

Botanical name: Matricaria recutita

Part used: flowers, essential oil

How to use: infusion – 25g dried flowers to 500ml boiling water taken in three equal daily doses; tincture – up to 5ml, three times a day; essential oil – 2–3 drops to 10ml of almond oil used in massage rubs

Both German chamomile *(Matricaria recutita)* and its relative Roman chamomile *(Chamaemelum nobile)* are among the most widely used of medicinal herbs. Their actions are very similar, with Roman chamomile having a slightly more bitter taste while German chamomile is slightly more anti-inflammatory and analgesic. Herbalists may have their individual favourites but the plants are extremely close in action and can be regarded as interchangeable in lay use.

The Greeks knew the herb as 'ground apple' (*kamai melon*) – so called because of its characteristic smell – and it is still used for ornamental lawns, giving a hint of apples when walked upon. To the Anglo-Saxons chamomile was *maythen*, one of the nine sacred herbs given to mankind by Woden and listed in the ninth-century poem the *Lacnunga*.

Both chamomiles are used as calming remedies for nervous upsets and in digestive problems mainly to ease abdominal cramps and clear gas. Externally the herb is widely used in creams for eczema, wounds, nappy rash, sore nipples and piles. The flowers are readily available in tea bags or sold loose for infusions and, although the flavour can be something of an acquired taste, chamomile tea is probably one of the most popular herbal drinks on the market.

The key chemical constituents are found in the deep blue essential oil, produced by steam distillation. This contains a substance called chamazulene produced in the distillation process which is highly anti-inflammatory. Chamomile extracts also contain a substance called apigenin which shows anti-anxiety activity (Viola *et al.*, 1995) while other trials have shown that inhaling chamomile oil tends to create a more positive mood while still having a sedative and calming action (Roberts and Williams, 1992).

Chamomile is also used in homoeopathy and Chamomilla 3X is a valuable standby for babies, used to treat both colic and teething. It is one of the safest herbs for children and babies and some mothers use weak infusions as a night-time drink to encourage restful sleep. The infusion can also be added to bath water to soothe over-excited infants.

Chamomile is ideal for easing anxiety states and would appear to have an uplifting effect on mood; it is readily available as the crude herb so is a good low-cost alternative to more exotic relaxation remedies.

Caution: chamomile can cause contact dermatitis. Rare cases of severe allergic reaction are known but these generally occur by those with existing pronounced allergies to members of the Compositae plant family.

NUTMEG

Botanical name: Myristica fragrans

Part used: seed, aril (mace)

How to use: Take up to 500mg in warm milk for insomnia or 3–5 drops of tincture as required for digestive problems

While Ayurvedic medicine regards nutmeg as one of the best medicines for calming the mind (Frawley and Lad, 1988) and promoting sound sleep, western herbalists tend to limit its use to digestive upsets and rheumatic disorders.

Nutmeg is the seed of a tree which originally grew only in the Moluccas or Spice Islands in the South Seas. The red covering of the seed (the aril) is known as mace and, like nutmeg, is widely used in cooking and flavourings. In folk medicine mace is made into an ointment used for rheumatism. Nutmeg was known to Avicenna as *jausiband* or 'nut of bands' and the tree was first brought to Europe from the Spice Islands by Portuguese sailors in around 1512. It rapidly gained the reputation of a cure-all and was widely eaten as a tonic.

Nutmeg contains myristicin (a phenol ether) which is hallucinogenic – a property which was soon discovered with the first report in 1576 of a 'pregnant English lady' who consumed 10–12 nuts and became, according to the herbalist Matthias L'Obel (1538–1616), 'deliriously inebriated'. She was possibly, unsuccessfully, trying to use nutmeg to procure an abortion – a property with which the herb was then erroneously endowed. It was – equally erroneously – acclaimed as a cure for the plague and 'sweating sickness'.

Nutmeg is a very warming remedy which also clears intestinal gas so it is effective for indigestion, intestinal colic and similar upsets. It is useful as a warming remedy for stomach chills which may be linked with watery diarrhoea or poor digestive function. It is also anti-emetic so effective for nausea and vomiting and is a popular addition for spicy winter drinks and mulled wines.

Nutmeg oil is also available and is used externally for

rheumatic pain and as an emergency treatment to dull toothache. In France drops of the oil are also taken internally in honey for digestive upsets or used for bad breath while in parts of the East, nutmeg oil is used as an aid for childbirth with pregnant mothers massaging the abdomen with a little oil (5 drops to 10ml of almond oil) for three weeks before the birth to help prepare for labour.

Nutmeg is known as *jatiphala* in Sanskrit and is often used in combination with cardamom and ginger for digestive problems or else mixed with buttermilk. While it is also effective at calming the mind, Ayurveda also describes it as *tamasic* – a heavy negative quality which in excess can lead to dullness of mind.

Nutmeg is known in Chinese medicine as *Rou Dou Kou* and has been used since at least the Tang Dynasty (*c.* AD600) mainly – as in the West – to warm the stomach and regulate *Qi* flow. *Rou Dou Kou* is also used for diarrhoea – especially the classic 'cock crow diarrhoea' which occurs on rising and can be related to *Qi* weakness.

Caution: a large dose (5g or more in a single dose) is hallucinogenic and can lead to convulsions, palpitations, coma and death.

JATAMANSI

Botanical name: Nardostachys grandiflora

Parts used: root, rhizome, essential oil

How to use: decoction – simmer 1 teaspoon of dried root in a cup of milk as a restoring tonic for tension and nervous upsets; tincture – up to 40 drops per dose

Spikenard – known as *jatamansi* in India – has been highly valued since biblical times: it is mentioned in the *Song of Solomon* and was regarded as a rejuvenating tonic by the Moghul emperors. The plant is related to valerian and shares its sedative properties, although it also has a more spiritual dimension – believed in

Ayurvedic medicine to promote awareness and strengthen the mind.

Jatamansi is believed to be the oil used to anoint Jesus at the Last Supper: As *St Mark's Gospel* has it: '. . .there came a woman having an alabaster box of ointment of spikenard very precious; and she brake the box, and poured it on his head' (Mark:14.3).

Jatamansi is now very rare in the wild and is listed as endangered by CITES (Convention on International Trade in Endangered Species of Wild Fauna and Flora); trade in the wild plant is only permitted by licence but alternative commercial cultivation is increasing and the herb grows readily in temperate climates.

Spikenard is not well researched: it is known to contain a volatile oil which is rich in borneol acetates but there has been very little attempt to assess its action or use the remedy in clinical trials. The oil is strongly anti-microbial as well as having sedative actions. It can be used in massage treatments for stress and nervous tension and can be added to external remedies for athlete's foot and other skin infections. In Indian folk medicine, *jatamansi* is used for a wide range of acute and chronic disorders including dysentery, consumption, bronchitis, smallpox, menstrual problems and digestive upsets. The aerial parts can be collected from garden-grown specimens and used in infusions as a gentle sedative and anti-bacterial for infections and fevers.

Jatamansi is mainly used in Ayurveda to balance the *doshas* (the essential substances that control health) and promote spiritual awareness as a rejuvenating tonic. It is both sedating to combat anxiety and spiritually uplifting adding a psychoactive dimension. It is also an effective cardiac tonic and respiratory stimulant.

Traditionally it is taken in milk decoction, popular in Ayurvedic therapeutics, but it can also be used in water decoctions or made into syrups for coughs and bronchitis. It is often combined with *gotu kola* which is believed to enhance its sedative action.

Fresh *jatamansi* is not easy to find in the West, unless in home cultivation, although the dried herb is available from Ayurvedic suppliers. The plant was always rare and expensive so would have been used only in small quantities.

LOTUS

Botanical name: Nelumbo nucifera

Parts used: seeds, root, leaves, stalk

How to use: up to 400mg of powdered seeds in capsules per dose; the leaves and stalk can be used in infusions

The lotus, or *padma*, is Indian's most sacred plant, with its symbolic unfolding petals suggesting growing spiritual awareness. As one early creation myth puts it:

> In the beginning were the waters. Matter readied itself. The sun glowed. And a lotus slowly opened, holding the universe on its golden pericarp.

In the East, the plant holds much the place of the rose in western Europe – a potent symbol of love and compassion. The lotus is sacred to Lakshmi, the goddess of prosperity, and it is believed to bring both material and spiritual wealth. It has been used medicinally since ancient Egyptian times and almost all parts are used in China for a wide range of ailments.

The seeds *(Lian Zi)* are mainly used as a tonic for the spleen and stomach to combat diarrhoea and stimulate the appetite. They are also used as a kidney tonic and a calming sedative to ease insomnia and palpitations. In India, where the plant is generally known as *padma,* the seeds are taken in powder format with rice as a tonic for the heart and reproductive organs. They are believed to help the heart *chakra* and to encourage devotion, aspiration and concentration, as well as improve speech and help reduce stammering. The inner seed parts – the plumules and radicles (*Lian Zi Xin*) – are classified as bitter and cold in Chinese medicine. They are used specifically to 'sedate the fire of the heart' – in Chinese theory this syndrome can be associated with fevers, irritability, high blood pressure, palpitations, insomnia, and restlessness. In Malaya the plumule is used for 'unlucky fever' or summer infections.

In China the flower stem (*Lian Fang*) is used to stop internal bleeding from gastric ulcers, abnormally heavy periods, blood in the stool, or post-partum haemorrhage. The stamens (*Lian Xu*) are believed to act on the heart and kidney. They are used to strengthen kidney energies where weakness is associated with frequent urination or premature ejaculation, and they will also stop nosebleeds and ease heavy menstrual bleeding.

The root and rhizome is most commonly used in India as a rejuvenating tonic specifically for problems affecting the first *chakra* (including diarrhoea, uterine disorders and haemorrhoids).

In China the rhizomes (*Ou Jie*) are used to stop bleeding – such as nosebleeds, spitting or coughing blood, blood in the urine and heavy menstrual bleeding. The leaves *(He Ye)* and leaf stems (*Lian Geng*) are mainly used in Chinese medicine as a cooling remedy for fevers associated with 'summer heat'. They are used as a spleen tonic for weaknesses associated diarrhoea and upsets following summer fevers.

Cautions: traditionally avoided in constipation and abdominal distension.

PASSION FLOWER

Botanical name: Passiflora incarnata

Parts used: aerial parts

How to use: take at night only for insomnia, repeating if need be once during the night or three times daily for anxiety or nervous tension; tincture – up to 3ml/60 drops per dose; capsules – up to 250mg per dose; infusion – 25g to 500ml water taken in three equal doses during the day

Passion flower takes its name not from any effect it may have on the emotions, but from the religious symbolism of its flowers: the three stigmas were taken to represent the nails of the Crucifixion, the five anthers were Christ's five wounds, while the ten petals represented the Apostles present at the time (Peter and Judas Iscariot having absented themselves).

The herb is known as maypop in North America and was traditionally used by the Houmas in Louisiana as a blood tonic while the Mayans regarded the crushed plant as helpful for swellings and used the decoction for ringworm. It was first described by a European botanist in the 1780s and by the nineteenth century had joined the herbal repertoire, initially as a remedy for epilepsy and later as a cure for insomnia.

Today, it is considered as an effective but gentle sedative and painkiller which will also reduce blood pressure. It is known to have a complex action on the nervous system (Speroni and Minghetti, 1981) due to some, as yet unidentified, constituents: those that have been isolated from the plant (including a group of alkaloids) appear to show little neuropharmacological activity. Passion flower is widely used in over-the-counter products for anxiety and nervous tension and is often combined with valerian or hops.

An infusion of the dried herb can also be helpful for period pain or tension headaches, and can be supportive for a number of other nervous conditions such as irritable bowel syndrome and irregular heart beats. The plant is slightly bitter and cooling so can also be helpful in feverish conditions.

Caution: avoid high doses in pregnancy.

JAMAICAN DOGWOOD

Botanical name: Piscidia piscipula

Part used: root bark

How to use: up to 5ml of tincture, three times daily

Although known as Jamaican dogwood this herb, which originates in Central America, Florida and the West Indies is unrelated to the more familiar *Cornus* pp. commonly grown as garden shrubs. The botanical name derives from the Latin *piscis*=fish and *caedere*=to kill: the plant was traditionally used by Native Americans as a fish poison (hence its alternative common name of Jamaican fish poison tree). Extracts from the plant were added to streams so stupefy the fish which then float to the surface and can be easily caught. The active principle is a group of chemicals called rotenoids, which stun the fish but leave the flesh untainted and still edible. Constituents include rotenone which has been well studied and is an effective insecticide and fish poison. This chemical has also been shown to have some anti-cancer activity although studies suggest that it is carcinogenic (Newell *et al.*, 1996).

The plant was introduced into Europe in the 1690s and was once popular as a conservatory ornamental, although it is now seldom grown here. Traditionally, it was used to prevent threatened miscarriage and ease labour pains and is still sometimes prescribed for period pain or after childbirth.

It is an effective painkiller and sedative and can be helpful for insomnia and anxiety-related disorders as well as neuralgia, muscular aches and pains and tension headaches. Although its constituents have been quite well investigated (Newell *et al.*, 1996; *PDR for Herbal Medicines*, 2000), there have been few clinical studies into its efficacy and some health care professionals advise that it should only be used by qualified practitioners. It may potentiate the sedative effects of other remedies.

It is often used in over-the-counter remedies in combination with valerian, black cohosh and skullcap.

PASQUE FLOWER

Botanical name: Pulsatilla vulgaris

Parts used: dried aerial parts

How to use: 10–50 drops of tincture, three times daily; up to 250mg dried herb in capsules

Pasque flowers are popular garden plants with bright purple petals, feathery leaves, and fluffy seed heads much loved by flower arrangers. The herb is a member of the buttercup family and various species are used in both European, North American and Chinese herbal tradition as well as in homoeopathy.

The common pasque flower (also known under the older botanical name of *Anemone pulsatilla*) is used as a mild sedative, anti-bacterial and analgesic which is also a specific for problems associated with the reproductive system. It is traditionally used for such disorders as inflammation of the ovaries, testes, or prostate gland, painful periods, and premenstrual syndrome. It is ideal for emotional upsets associated with the menopause and can also be used in childhood diseases – especially mumps and measles.

The herb is also often recommended for hearing disorders – used in combination with ginkgo or hawthorn – and some believe that it can be used for certain clinical mental problems (Bartram, 1995). The plant is poorly researched although animal studies have confirmed action on the female reproductive organs and sedative properties (Newell *et al.*, 1996).

It combines well with other relaxants: a combination of pasque flower, passion flower and Jamaican dogwood is a popular combination for anxiety, tension, insomnia and also hyperactivity in children. It also works well with skullcap and lemon balm.

Caution: the fresh herb should not be used as it contains a toxic chemical called protoanemonin which breaks down to harmless substances when the plant is dried; it should be avoided in pregnancy.

DAN SHEN

Botanical name: Salvia miltiorrhiza

Parts used: root and rhizome

How to use: use in a decoction made from brewing 15g of dried herb in two cups of water for twenty minutes, strain the liquid and take in a single daily dose

Dan Shen – Chinese sage – is one of China's most important heart and blood tonics which has been shown in clinical trials to help both heart disease and problems with cerebral circulation. It is traditionally described as 'invigorating' the blood to combat congealed or stagnant blood.

'Stagnant blood' in a traditional Chinese disease syndrome description for conditions where the flow of blood is blocked or the blood becomes static. This may be the result of external pathogens, be caused by inappropriate treatment of haemorrhage, by traumatic injury, by stagnation of *Qi*, or – in women – by retention of the lochia following childbirth (Yanchi, 1988). Stagnant blood is characterised by a fixed pain which is not eased by either hot compresses or ice packs and typical signs include purplish skin, dark purple lips and dry scaly skin.

In modern medicine conditions like thrombosis, local ischaemia, menstrual problems, certain heart disorders or haemorrhage might all be classified in TCM as aspects of congealed blood.

Dan Shen is the herb of choice for treating heart problems such as angina pectoris and coronary heart disease which may be associated with stagnant blood. In Chinese theory the liver is involved with regulating the menstrual cycle so it is no surprise that *Dan Shen* (which affects the liver meridian) is a key herb for stagnant blood problems in the lower abdomen – the sorts of disorders which in the West we would term dysmenorrhoea (period pain) or amenorrhoea (absence of periods). Because it is also cooling *Dan Shen* is used for problems associated with heat and toxins in the blood which the Chinese would see as the cause of boils and skin ulcers.

Significantly, too, because the heart is also associated with the spirit and mental activity, then the combined cooling aspect and heart focus of *Dan Shen* make it suitable as a sedative or tranquilliser given for insomnia, irritability and palpitations.

While these attributes date back long before the days of chemical analysis and modern pathology, modern trials do suggest that *Dan Shen* is effective in all these ways. As well as its action on the circulatory system, *Dan Shen* has been shown to lower blood sugar and blood cholesterol levels, increase metabolism and stimulate the immunity system. Decoctions of the herb have been shown in animal studies to improve coronary blood flow and combat the effects of myocardial infarction, dilate the coronary blood vessels and peripheral blood vessels, so helping to reduce blood pressure, increase blood flow – especially in the micro-circulation (Chang and But, 1986) – and it will also enhance the activity of other cardiotonic herbs to improve cardiac output (Zhu *et al.*, 1987).

There have been a number of studies in this area in recent years which have demonstrated that *Dan Shen* can be very effective for combating a range of heart and circulatory disorders. (Bensky and Gamble, 1986; Foster and Chongxi, 1992). Other studies have shown how *Dan Shen* injections can reduce mortality from heart attacks from 39 per cent to 13 per cent if treatment is given within twenty-four hours, and it has also been used in a similar way in combination with other herbs with good results (Keji, 1981; Guo *et al.*, 1983),

The herb has also been used in trials involving patients suffering from cerebral atherosclerosis – a common cause of dizziness and confusion in the elderly. In a small-scale test, 26 from a total of 42 patients were deemed 'cured' while a further 11 showed significant improvement using a range of remedies selected to match the likely cause of their problems (Li *et al.*, 1987).

As well as its established uses in heart and menstrual problems, research has also shown that *Dan Shen* is protective for both heart and liver, reduces blood pressure, makes a useful wound herb and is anti-coagulant and anti-bacterial. Tests have shown that it will combat a variety of bacteria and it shows some anti-cancer activity in laboratory experiments (Bone, 1996).

Its action on the heart can make it a valuable sedative remedy in some cases while it may also be useful for confused elderly patients by helping to improve cerebral circulation.

SANDALWOOD

Botanical name: Santalum album

Parts used: Inner heartwood, essential oil

How to use: traditionally taken in India as a powder (up to 500mg per dose) stirred in ghee (clarified butter) or milk; the oil is used in massage (5 drops to 15ml of almond oil)

Sandalwood – known as *chandana* in Sanskrit – is one of Ayurveda's most popular remedies – used to cool and calm the body and mind, awaken the intelligence and open the 'third eye' to increase devotion and meditation. The wood is often burned as incense and the oil features in many Hindu rituals. The oil has a sweet, woody, rose-like scent and is used in perfumery while aromatherapists often combine it with rose, neroli or benzoin oils to produce a calming, sedative and anti-depressant massage. It is also a reputed sexual tonic to combat impotence and poor libido so is sometimes called 'lover's oil'.

The tree is native to India but has been grossly over-exploited both for its wood and oil and is now classified as in danger of extinction in the wild in the medium term. The tree takes up to forty years to reach maturity and since the oil can only be distilled from the heartwood production almost inevitably destroys the tree. It is illegal to export the wood from India although a lucrative smuggling trade exists; unless the source is known and has been ethically harvested it is, sadly, best to avoid using sandalwood.

The wood is used in decoctions for fevers, inflammations and as a circulatory or digestive stimulant. It is known as *Tan Xiang* in China and is believed to normalise energy flows to stomach and spleen, to stimulate the digestion and relieve pain. Sandalwood is also strongly antiseptic and anti-bacterial and can be used as a wash or made into a paste for external sores. The oil can be used in massage for urinary problems, including cystitis, and digestive upsets with abdominal discomfort. It can be added to warm compresses for dry skin, itching and irritation and also added to rosewater as a lotion for acne.

A few drops to the brow *chakra* (third eye) can improve concentration and cool the body in fevers and thirst.

Studies have shown that sandalwood has some anti-viral properties (Conway, 2001) and is a specific for *Herpes simplex* – the virus responsible for cold sores and genital herpes.

Cautions: Do not take the essential oil internally.

SKULLCAP

Botanical name: Scutellaria lateriflora

Parts used: aerial parts

How to use: tincture – up to 4ml/80 drops, three times a day; infusion 25g to 500ml of boiling water taken in three equal doses daily

Virginian skullcap was first introduced into Europe in the eighteenth century and was used as a treatment for rabies – hence its alternative name of 'mad dog'. It was used by the Cherokee to encourage menstruation and also to treat diarrhoea and breast pains. Today, it is considered mainly as a sedative and nervine by western herbalists but may also be used to reduce fevers, calm the foetus, and stimulate the digestion.

Like all skullcaps, the Virginian variety takes its name from the dish-shaped seed pods, while its botanical name is derived from the growing pattern of the flowers which appear on only one side of the stem. Virginian skullcap grows easily in British gardens and will self-seed enthusiastically – to the point where it can become invasive. European skullcap species (such as *S. galericulata*) have very similar properties although there is little tradition of using them in herbal medicine.

As well as its sedating properties, skullcap is now also known to be anti-bacterial, to lower both blood pressure and blood cholesterol levels and to ease spasmodic pains. Drinking skullcap tea can encourage relaxation and combat anxiety and nervous tension. Skullcap tea can also be useful to soothe pre-menstrual tension and menstrual cramps.

Like other North American plants, the herb is not especially well researched although one study (Murch *et al.*, 1997) found the chemical melatonin to be present in the plant. Melatonin – a hormone which in responsible for inducing hibernation in some mammals – has become popular in recent years in supplements as a remedy for both insomnia and jet lag. Skullcap had one of the highest melatonin levels found in the plants investigated and this may account for some of skullcap's sedative action.

There is also one reported clinical trial of the use of skullcap extract for treating cerebral thrombosis and paralysis following stroke. Over all some 88 per cent of those given the herb reported some degree of improvement (Peigen and Keji, 1987).

WOOD BETONY

Botanical name: Stachys officinalis

Parts used: aerial parts

How to use: infusion – 25g of dried herb to 500ml of boiling water taken in three equal doses daily; tincture – up to 5ml, three times a day

Although wood betony tends to be rather neglected these days, it was one of the most important healing plants in the Anglo-Saxon repertoire: no fewer than twenty-nine uses of it are known and as well as recommending it for a range of physical diseases, it was a popular amulet herb used well into the Middle Ages – tied on to the arm with red wool to ward off evil or ill humours. As late as 1526 *The Grete Herball* was recommending it 'for them that be ferful', while William Turner, in 1551, advises that it will heal 'them that are mad' and John Gerard (1597) gives a very long list of applications concluding that 'it maketh a man to pisse well'.

The herb is an attractive one for the garden with bright cerise flowers in late summer to autumn. It is mainly used these days as a nervine and sedative for headaches and nervous debility and it makes a very pleasant-tasting tea. It is also a good anti-catarrhal herb and, taken in a tea or tincture, can help reduce the discomfort of sinusitis and severe nasal congestion. Betony is also slightly bitter and so helps to stimulate digestive function. It will also help encourage blood flow to the brain and can be useful in the elderly where restricted cerebral circulation often leads to mental confusion; this can erroneously be interpreted as a sign of dementia.

Culpeper, in 1653, stressed that it 'preserves the liver and bodies of men from epidemical diseases and from witchcraft' and it certainly has an affinity with the liver – ideal for poor or sluggish digestion, and as a general stimulant. It can be especially helpful for menopausal problems and is ideal in childbirth to encourage contractions and relax the mother.

The herb is not especially well researched although studies have identified a variety of constituents including bitter iridoids which may account for its digestive function. It is, however, an effective and pleasant-tasting sedative to ease anxiety and one which can also stimulate cerebral circulation to combat confusion in the elderly.

Cautions: although helpful during labour, wood betony should be avoided in pregnancy as it is a uterine stimulant.

LINDEN

Botanical name: Tilia cordata

Part used: flowers

How to use: infusion – 25g of dried herb to 500ml boiling water taken in three equal doses daily; tincture – up to 4ml/80 drops, three times a day

Flowers from the European lime or linden tree can be collected in late summer to provide a convenient, soothing remedy that can also help combat high blood pressure. The herb is believed to counter the build-up of fatty deposits in blood vessels that can lead to arteriosclerosis or 'hardening of the arteries'. In France, linden is known as *tilleul* and is one of the most popular of after-dinner tisanes.

The plant was regarded by medieval herbalists as hot and drying, so it was recommended for headaches caused by cold and was also used for dizziness and epilepsy. Linden is mildly sedative, encourages perspiration and will also ease muscle spasms and cramps. Although we now use only the flowers medicinally, the leaves were once made into ointments for swellings or sores and used in mouthwashes for minor gum infections.

The flowers combine well with lemon balm for nervous tension and anxiety or can be mixed with hawthorn flowers for high blood pressure. Because it is both calming and reduces blood pressure herb, lime flowers are ideal for those suffering from high blood pressure which is related to stress. It can also be suitable for digestive upsets associated with nervous tension and in feverish colds or influenza.

Linden is not especially well researched although some anti-fungal activity has been noted (Guerin and Reveillere, 1984).

As a sedative and diaphoretic it is especially useful for those suffering from stress-related high blood pressure and other cardio-vascular disorders. The tea is pleasant to take and widely available in tea bags,

VALERIAN

Botanical name: Valeriana officinalis

Part used: root.

How to use: capsules – up to 400mg per dose, three times daily; tincture up to 4ml/80 drops per dose, three times daily; maceration – prepared by soaking 25g of dried herb to 500ml of cold water overnight, taken in three equal doses

Valerian is often described as nature's tranquilliser – a calming nervine without the side effects of comparable orthodox drugs: it does not cause drowsiness and so is one of the few sedatives that can be safely taken to steady the nerves before a driving test, for example.

The botanical name is derived from the Latin *valere* which means 'well being' and the herb has been used as a sedative throughout Europe for more than 2,000 years. It has a distinctive, rather unpleasant smell and was aptly called *phu* by the second century Roman physician Galen. Cats, however, love it and will roll ecstatically in the growing plants.

The rhizomes and roots are used medicinally and are harvested in the autumn and spring. The plant is tall (up to 140cm) with densely packed, pale pink flowers and is an easy plant to cultivate in domestic gardens but should not be confused with American valerian, often sold by garden centres, which has red flowers.

The plant has been extensively researched over the past few decades initially with the aim of identifying the aromatic oils which give the characteristic smell. This varies between the fresh plant and older, dried specimens and it is now known that the active chemicals in the plant oxidise and change significantly with ageing. More than thirty compounds have been identified in the essential oil and among the more significant are isovalerate, valerenic acid, and valeranone.

At first it was thought that the essential oil was primarily responsible for the plant's sedative action but during the 1960s researchers found very little correlation between that and the chemicals then identified. Further work followed (Thies, 1968) and eventually a group of compounds collectively labelled as 'valepotriates' were identified: they included valtrate, *l*-acevaltrate and dihydrovaltrate. Over thc next twenty years many similar compounds were identified and studied, but again, evidence that these actually have sedative properties has been scant.

The valepotriates are also present in quite low quantities (around 1.2 per cent, but, despite their scarcity, they have been extensively studied and show various properties including anti-tumour activity. These chemicals develop as the plant dries so tinctures made from fresh and dried valerian roots can have quite different chemical compositions. Some suggest that the vale-potriates have a slightly more depressant effect on the nervous system while the fresh plant is more sedating.

Valerian has also long been known to contain alkaloids (Torssell and Wahlberg, 1967) these include valeranine and actinidine which have an effect on the chemistry of the body's neurotransmitters.

Having identified the various active chemicals, the researchers were keen to apportion sedative activity to them in the hope of identifying any chemicals which could be synthesised to form new drugs. However, valerian has proved rather more complicated and elusive with its tranquillising action derived from a combination of the chemicals found in the essential oil, the valepotriates and the degradation products of the valepotriates that are formed in the tincture as it ages.

Studies have also shown that these chemicals are good muscle relaxants (see Morazzoni and Bombardelli, 1995, for an extensive review) with no side-effects or toxicity reported even when the herb has been extensively tested on pregnant laboratory animals. In one widely reported case (Wiley, 1995), a woman attempted to commit suicide by swallowing around fifty capsules, each containing 470mg of powdered valerian root, which is around ten times the maximum recommended dosage. After half an hour she complained of tiredness, abdominal cramps, tightness in the chest, tremors in the hands and feet, and lightheadedness. However, liver function remained normal and after twenty-four hours all symptoms had resolved.

There have also been a number of clinical trials involving valerian which have demonstrated its efficacy at easing anxiety, menopausal emotional upsets and insomnia. Valerian can also help to relax smooth muscle so can ease the sort of stomach cramps associated with nervous tension and can be valuable in some types of high blood pressure.

One trial (Leatherwood *et al.*, 1982) involving 128 people, for example, showed dramatic improvements in sleep quality among poor or irregular sleepers as well as some benefit for the good sleepers involved in the trial. Dosage was 400mg of a water-based valerian extract taken at night. In another double-blind study (Lindahl and Lindwall, 1989) volunteers with self-reported sleep difficulties were given a valerian extract standardised for its essential oil content. Some 44 per cent of the subjects reported a perfect night's sleep as a result while in total 89 per cent claimed improved sleep. Additional studies have shown that between two and four weeks of valerian use may be needed before the herb takes effect (Schulz *et al.*, 1997).

Most of these clinical trials have used up to 600mg of valerian extract in a daily dose which is equivalent to around 2.4g of crude dried root and rhizome.

While most of these trials have focused on sleep patterns, one with forty-eight volunteers placed under experimental 'social stress' conditions (Kohnen and Oswald, 1988) showed that quite low doses of valerian root extract (100mg) reduced subjective feelings of tension and made the volunteers generally feel better, although there was little physiological evidence of any change in body activity.

Some researchers and practitioners argue that even with the limited number of studies completed so far, there is plenty of evidence to confirm valerian's efficacy, at least as an insomnia remedy. However, critics – which have included the official United States *Pharmacopoeia* – suggest that the evidence is scanty. The official monograph on valerian from the European Scientific Co-operative on Phytotherapy (ESCOP, 1997) recommends the herb for 'tenseness, restlessness and irritability with difficulty in falling asleep' and gives the recommended dose as 2–3 g of the root taken as a cup of infusion or 1–3ml of a 1:5 tincture up to three times daily.

In spite of these official doubts, valerian is probably the most widely used over-the-counter herbal sedative on the market today. It is included in very many proprietary products marketed for anxiety and insomnia and is also prescribed by herbalists for a variety of heart conditions. It is popular in proprietary remedies targeted at menopausal women and for anxiety associated with premenstrual syndrome and period pain. The herb also shows some anti-bacterial action, it will help to clear gas from the digestive track and ease spasmodic cramps.

Valerian tea – best made by cold water maceration rather than hot infusion – can be a useful household remedy for nervous irritability, tension headaches, menopausal problems, bronchial spasm and smoker's cough. A strong maceration of the fresh root can be added to bath water to make a relaxing bath when suffering from nervous exhaustion – although the smell is not to everyone's taste.

Anecdotal evidence also suggests that valerian can have unexpected and adverse effects on some people – exciting rather than calming and possibly causing headaches – so its use needs some caution initially. Long-term use can also sometimes lead to insomnia so it is best to have regular breaks in therapy of two to three weeks after three months and the herb should not be taken for more than six months continuously.

Valerian has proven efficacy in treating both anxiety and insomnia – and as at least one clinical study has shown, even though its action is not well understood, the herb does bestow a 'feel-good factor' in stressful situations.

Mostly energy-giving

Tonic herbs are found in all cultures and have a long history as energy-giving remedies. Ayurvedic tonics, as discussed earlier (Chapter 3) can have both spiritual and physical aspects.

Chinese tonics tend to focus on revitalising various aspects of *Qi* – often understood in the West as our inner energy level but actually a more complex substance which in Chinese theory comes in a wide variety of types. Its main characteristic is motion: the activity of life. Some scholars suggest that as many as thirty-two different varieties of *Qi*, each with its own specific function and characteristics, have been described in Chinese texts over the past 2,500 years with changing emphasis and terminology over the centuries adding to the confusion.

Qi is basically a mixture of energies derived from the food we eat and the air we breathe, plus an element inherited from our parents which is with us from birth. These raw ingredients then combine and are transformed in a variety of ways to make the different sorts of *Qi* which circulate in the body. Tonic remedies can be focused on these various sorts of *Qi* – such as milk vetch which strengthens *Wei Qi* (the defence energy that protects us against external attack and can be equated with our western concept of an immune system).

Use of tonic herbs in China goes back to the early Taoists. They believed that the ideal way of life to achieve prosperity, longevity and immortality was to encourage 'virtue'. Virtue meant conforming to nature and living in harmony with all things. Herbal tonics were part of this 'cultivation of the Way' helping to integrate physical and spiritual growth and encourage determination to follow the path of virtue. Many of these herbs are described as 'longevity tonics' today.

Herbal energy tonics are so familiar in the West that we tend to ignore them: tea and coffee are rich in stimulating alkaloids (theobromine and caffeine) which provide a short-term boost to our energies. The uplifting effect of drinking a cup of tea or coffee when you are tired or over-worked is appreciated by all – yet we would rarely put these herbs in the same category as ginseng or guarana. While caffeine-based herbs provide only a superficial energy tonic, others have a more deep-seated effect. Rosemary contains a chemical called borneol which acts as a powerful stimulant to the nervous system to overcome fatigue. This same compound is also found in other common culinary herbs such as sage and thyme both of which can be used in stimulating and energy-giving teas.

In general, tonic herbs should be avoided during acute illness and infection as their strengthening action can also energise invading micro-organisms.

ALOE VERA

Botanical name: Aloe spp.

Part used: sap, leaves

How to use: sap – generally 10–20ml, three times day; capsules – up to 1.5g daily; tincture (purgative) – up to 40 drops per dose, three times a day

Aloe vera has become a fashionable and popular over-the-counter remedy for a wide range of ills in recent years. The whole aloe plant is used as a strong purgative: 'bitter aloes', once a household standby for constipation, is a leaf extract made from various species of aloe.

Aloe is a tropical African plant which has been used medicinally since ancient Greek and Roman times. The plant reached the West Indies with the slave trade in the sixteenth century and has been widely cultivated there ever since – hence such common names as Barbados or Curaçao aloes. In the West, the juice has traditionally been regarded as a soothing wound herb, although in Ayurvedic medicine it is treated as a restorative tonic.

The whole leaf is a bitter purgative and digestive stimulant and common remedy in over-the-counter products for constipation: an extract 'bitter aloes' was once standard on pharmacists' shelves as a laxative and is generally made from a combination of various species of aloe. The same liquid was popularly painted on children's fingers to stop them sucking or biting nails.

'Aloe vera' is the name commonly given to the mucilaginous sap obtained from such species as *A. barbadensis* and this was largely used externally in the West as a wound healer and to relieve burns and skin inflammations including eczema and thrush. This gel, usually cold-pressed from the leaves is now also made into a variety of popular tonic remedies promoted as energy restoratives and pick-you-ups.

In Ayurvedic tradition, the sap is used as a restorative for the female reproductive system and as a tonic for the liver and spleen. It comes into the 'nutritive tonic' category and is often combined with *shatavari* – also a specific female tonic. It is more palatable if mixed with apple juice or water: use two teaspoons of the sap with a pinch of turmeric mixed with 2–3 teaspoons of water or apple juice.

The plant grows well in the UK as a house plant but will generally not survive out of doors for long. Although it looks like a succulent, aloe is more closely related to the lily family so needs plenty of water. The gel is easy to collect by simply breaking open a leaf and scraping out the sap; alternatively fresh leaves can be split and applied directly to wounds and inflammations. It can usefully be grown on a kitchen windowsill as a convenient first-aid standby for minor burns. The sap can also be used on eczema and can help with fungal infections such as ringworm and thrush.

Cautions: avoid in pregnancy as it is strongly purgative; high doses of leaf extracts may cause vomiting. Some commercial preparations of sap are polluted with high levels of aloin – a purgative chemical found in the leaves which may cause nausea and diarrhoea.

SHATAVARI

Botanical name: Asparagus racemosus

Parts used: root

How to use: traditionally taken in a decoction made from milk (25g per 500ml) or as ground powder (up to 1g per dose) stirred into a cup of hot milk or mixed with ghee (clarified butter) or honey

A close relative of our familiar western vegetable asparagus, *shatavari* is one of Ayurveda's most important rejuvenative tonics. The name *shatavari* means 'who possesses a hundred husbands' and the herb is believed in India to have an extremely beneficial effect on the female reproductive organs.

Shatavari is primarily used for any debility associated with the female sexual organs including infertility, menopausal problems and following hysterectomy. It is also regarded as a soothing demulcent for the digestive and respiratory systems used for dry coughs, fevers associated with thirst, pleurisy, sunstroke, and inflammatory digestive problems such as dysentery. The herb is taken as a milk stimulant for lactating mothers and is believed to increase fertility. In Ayurveda it is described as '*sattvic*'– a quality associated with light, perception, intelligence and harmony which it is believed to promote. In China the roots are mainly used as cooling remedy to clear heat and replenish body fluids, given for symptoms of kidney energy weakness, such as night sweats and impotence.

Cautions: traditionally avoided in cases of diarrhoea and coughs caused by common colds.

HUANG QI

Botanical name: Astragalus membranaceus

Parts used: root

How to use: tincture – up to 3ml/60 drops, three times a day; decoction – up to 45g in 750ml of water taken in three equal doses; capsules – up to 600mg daily; traditionally the fried root is simply chewed like a snack

Huang Qi is an important energy tonic traditionally used in China for younger people while Korean ginseng is considered better for the over-forties. The two herbs are also frequently used together as a general tonic. The name translates literally as 'yellow leader' reflecting both the colour of the root and the plant's importance as a major tonic remedy. The herb is included in the famous herbal attributed to Shen Nong – the legendary founder of Chinese herbal medicine – where it is listed among the 'superior' remedies. The plant is known in the West as milk vetch and can occasionally be found in health food shops under this name although it is more commonly labelled as 'astragalus'.

Huang Qi is believed to strengthen defence energy (*Wei Qi*) which in Chinese tradition is the body's protection from external 'evils'. Modern research has confirmed that the plant is an important anti-bacterial and immune stimulant and it has been used in AIDS treatments and also as an immune tonic in cancer patients undergoing chemotherapy. Because of its strong immune-stimulating action astragalus is often promoted as a cancer preventative and can also be useful for those suffering from recurrent infections.

The plant is also used as a heart tonic to combat heart disease and stimulate the blood circulation. It will reduce blood pressure and also lower blood sugar levels.

As well as its energy stimulating action, *Huang Qi* is also regarded as a blood tonic and is sometimes used in China with *Dang Gui* in blood deficiency associated with prolonged bleeding – as in heavy menstrual bleeding. Astragalus also acts as a nerve and digestion stimulant and is particularly useful for any condition which causes immune suppression such as chemotherapy or radiotherapy.

It can be used with both Korean and Siberian ginseng to improve stamina or with *Dan Shen* to combat ageing and help the heart.

The herb has been extensively researched in recent years although which constituents are key is still unclear. It contains a group of triterpenoid saponins which are known to increase anti-bacterial activity and stimulate the immune system while various plant sterols may be associated with its tonic action (Bone, 1996).

SAFFRON

Botanical name: Crocus sativus

Parts used: flower stigma

How to use: although expensive a little goes a long way. Use a pinch in cooking or simmer a pinch in milk as a decoction

Known as *nagakeshara* in Sanskrit, saffron is used in India as a blood tonic, stimulant and aphrodisiac. It is a potent – but expensive – tonic for the circulation, and female reproductive system. Saffron is very restorative and in Ayurveda is used to strengthen feelings of love, devotion and compassion.

The herb is the *karcom* of the Hebrews – mentioned in the *Song of Solomon* (iv.14) and its use was certainly widespread in ancient Greek times – Homer sings of 'the saffron morn'. Saffron is traditionally used to dye monks robes in Buddhism and in the East its aroma has been described as 'perfect ambrosia' (Grieve, 1931). The herb has been imported into the UK for centuries although it was once extensively cultivated in East Anglia – especially around Saffron Walden. Until the 1920s it was still used in British folk medicine for measles and other childhood ailments.

The cost is, howver, high – understandable when one considers that it is said that 125,000 crocus stigmas make up 1kg of saffron.

Saffron is believed in Ayurvedic theory to enhance the efficacy of other tonic herbs so a pinch is often added to other remedies. It is used with *shatavari* or *Dang Gui* as a tonic for the female reproductive organs and function especially at the menopause. Saffron is also believed to help the digestion with a pinch added as a spice to help energise food.

In western terms the herb is carminative – clearing intestinal gas to ease gastric upsets and indigestion – and is also regarded as an expectorant suitable for dry coughs, bronchitis and whooping cough.

It has been used in the West for insomnia and hysterical states although – largely because of its price – tends nowadays to be confined to culinary use.

GOTU KOLA

Botanical name: Centella asiatica

Parts used: aerial parts

How to use: powder/capsules – up to 500mg per dose, three times daily; dried herb – infusions made from 20g of herb to 500ml water taken in three equal daily does; tincture – up to 80 drops/ 4ml per dose. three times daily; a paste made of the powder is used externally for eczema and skin sores

Indian pennywort or *gotu kola* is known as *brahmi* in Sanskrit as it increases knowledge of *Brahman*, the supreme reality. It is one of the most important rejuvenative remedies (*rasayana karma*) in Ayurveda.

These types of tonics are believed to help combat ageing and senility and will improve the memory. They are also believed to enhance mental clarity and spiritual awareness helping to revitalise the brain and nervous system. In Ayurvedic theory *gotu kola* is believed to be a specific tonic for *pitta* (fire/bile). This is one of the three fundamental substances or '*doshas*' which Ayurvedic theory believes must be held in balance if the body is to remain healthy. While tonifying *pitta*, *gotu kola* also helps to reduce any excesses of the *vata* (air/wind) and *kapha* (damp/phlegm) *doshas,* and so is regarded as calming and an important aid for spiritual renewal.

The herb has been known in Europe for generations and tends to be used for more physical disorders such as skin problems, poor circulation and rheumatic aches and pains. It was once used for severe conditions such as leprosy and syphilis and is a powerful blood cleanser to clear toxins from the system. *Gotu kola* has also been used by western herbalists for nervous problems and depression and is sometimes given to help strengthen the nervous system in Parkinson's disease. It is anti-inflammatory and will also stimulate the immune system, and is therefore a useful herb for infections.

Among its active constituents are an alkaloid (hydrocotyline), triterpene saponins and phenolic glycosides – although how these account for the herb's action has yet to be fully investigated.

Gotu kola has long had a reputation for improving the memory and increasing mental awareness – a factor confirmed in a 1992 study (Nalini *et al.*, 1992) which demonstrated that the herb could improve memory in laboratory rats. The animals were fed extracts for fourteen days before being set a trial task to learn. Behaviour retention in the *gotu-kola*-fed rats was up to sixty times as good as the control animals. *Gotu kola* is the preferred forage choice of the Indian elephant – which, as they say, 'never forgets'.

Two studies (summarised in *Herbalgram,* 1993) have also shown that *gotu kola* can improve IQ and behaviour in mentally retarded children. The research suggests that the action is due to an effect the plant appears to have on the neurotransmitters, especially dopamine and serotonin. These neurotransmitters are also involved in Parkinson's disease, which helps to explain the plant's traditional use in easing symptoms of this chronic condition. In one study extracts of fresh leaves were used in doses of up to 16g per kg body weight. This would be equivalent in an adult subject of more than 1kg of fresh leaf per dose. No side effects were noticed and the researchers simply added that none would be expected as the plant is a well established food source in many parts of Asia (eaten by humans as well as elephants).

However, other reports suggest that the herb can cause severe headaches if more than six fresh leaves are eaten; since other plants are also known as *brahmi* in the Indian sub-continent there could be some confusion in species that is clouding the literature. In India fresh leaves of *gotu kola* are given to children to combat digestive disorders including dysentery and it is mixed with oil as a scalp rub to stimulate hair growth. *Gotu kola* is traditionally taken in milk decoction or can be mixed with *ghee* (clarified butter) as a revitalising remedy for the spirit. It is also used with basil as a cooling remedy in fevers and food poisoning.

Other studies (Boughton, 1998) have shown that *gotu kola* can be especially helpful in the elderly for circulatory problems helping to improve the efficiency of the veins and accelerate healing in varicose ulcers. Research in the 1990s suggest that the plant could reduce fertility so is best avoided by those hoping to conceive. A recent study (Bradwein *et al.*, 2000) has also shown that *gotu kola* can cause a significant reduction in feelings of anxiety, fearfulness and nervousness: a study of forty healthy subjects were subjected to an artificial stimulant to test the 'acoustic startle response' (ASR) – the physiological reaction to a loud noise. Those taking *gota kola* were significantly less startled.

Gotu kola has a relaxing effect but will also increase mental awareness. Despite the conflicting reports high doses do seem to be well tolerated and although it needs to be used with caution in pregnancy it is comparatively safe in long term regular dose – it is easy to make as an infusion and, unlike some herbs, it also tastes quite pleasant.

Cautions: avoid high doses in pregnancy and completely in epilepsy.

DANG SHEN

Botanical name: Codonopsis pilosula

Parts used: root

How to use: generally taken as a decoction (up to 15g per day); also available as tinctures (up to 3ml/60 drops three times daily)

Dang Shen is an important Chinese '*yin*' tonic. In traditional Chinese medicine the Taoist concepts of '*yin*' and '*yang*' are applied to both bodily organs and energy states and both aspects must be in balance to maintain health. '*Yin* deficiency' commonly effects the lungs, stomach, liver and kidneys. *Yin* tonics are used to combat these weaknesses and also help to increase body fluids – moistening tissues and having a laxative effect to help clear phlegm by making it less sticky and heavy.

Modern research has shown that *yin* tonics also tend to reduce high blood pressure and cholesterol levels. Typical symptoms of *yin* deficiency include: feverishness and night sweats; and thirst and dry mouth. The problem is also associated with debility following a long illness.

Dang Shen is often used as a rather less expensive alternative to Korean ginseng. The herb is considered to be gentler and more *yin* in character than ginseng and is traditionally taken by nursing mothers. Gentle it may be, but is still an effective *Qi* tonic for spleen, stomach,and lungs ideal for deficiency ailments characterised by tiredness, loss of appetite, aching limbs, palpitations, chronic coughs and shortness of breath.

As well as its tonic action, *Dang Shen* is also used in Chinese medicine to provide protection against stomach ulcers – often associated with excessive stress allowing the *Heliobacter pylori* bacterium, which can cause the ulcers, to get out of control. Recent studies (Shan *et al.*, 1999) have also shown that the herb can ease the symptoms of irritable bowel syndrome – another disorder often related to stress. Sufferers took high doses of the plant (fifteen capsules containing 600mg daily) for four months with significant improvements reported.

Dang Shen is an ingredient in a popular Chinese remedy called 'Change of Season Soup' (which also contains *Huang Qi*) used whenever there are major shifts in the weather to help the body adapt more easily to new conditions.

KOLA

Botanical name: Cola nitida

Parts used: seeds

How to use: powdered in capsules up to 3g per dose or in decoctions (up to 1/2 teaspoon per cup)

Kola contains up to 2.5 per cent of caffeine with traces of theobromine making it a rather more effective stimulant than coffee (which contains up to around 0.3 per cent caffeine). The tree originates in Africa where – rather like khat and coca leaves – the seeds were traditionally chewed to allay feelings of hunger and combat fatigue.

Like other caffeine sources, kola essentially provides a short-term energy boost rather than acting as a more deep-seated energy tonic. Caffeine stimulates the central nervous system to give a short-term uplift in performance. It also acts as a stimulant for the heart (hence coffee's association with palpitations) and the circulatory system.

It was used in the original Coca-Cola recipe – the 'coca' being provided by cocaine leaves. Tablets containing 5g of kola, called 'Forced March', were regularly issued to troops in the early years of the twentieth century to provide an energy boost. It is sometimes combined with saw palmetto and damiana for male sexual problems or with skullcap for depression and nervous debility.

Cautions: because of its high caffeine content kola can be associated with sleep disturbances, nervous restlessness and over-excitability. It should be avoided by anyone with high blood pressure and always used with moderation.

SIBERIAN GINSENG

Botanical name: Eleutherococcus senticosus

Part used: root

How to use: tincture – up to 20ml three times day; capsules up to 600mg three times daily.

Siberian ginseng belongs to one of the oldest known plant families, the Araliacaea, and has been used in Chinese medicine for around 2,000 years. It was traditionally regarded as a warming herb to strengthen the sinews and bones and to improve energy and blood flows, especially in the elderly. Its Chinese name, *Wu Jia Pi*, means 'bark of five additions' – reminding us that the Chinese used only the root bark, not the whole root as in the West.

The plant was 'discovered' by western scientists in the 1930s in Russia and subsequently used extensively by Soviet athletes to increase stamina and enhance performance. It has since been well researched and is known to stimulate the immune and circulatory systems and also help regulate blood pressure and lower blood sugar levels.

Key constituents include a group of plant sterols and triterpenoid saponins which are believed to account for its immune stimulating activity.

As the Soviet researchers discovered back in the 1930s, Siberian ginseng is especially effective at increasing stamina and helping the body cope more efficiently with both physical and mental stresses. Researchers (Brekhman and Dardymov, 1969) coined the term 'adaptagen' to describe this sort of action. Studies (Fulder, 1980) have shown that Siberian ginseng can increase stamina by up to 70 per cent and can also reduce the pathological signs of stress – such as enlarged adrenal glands – found in laboratory animals subjected to such excesses. It can also improve resistance to cold, heat, trauma, surgery and various toxins (Brekhman and Dardymov, 1969).

The herb does have its downside, however. Some studies have found that laboratory rats fed excessive amounts of Siberian ginseng display abnormally aggressive behaviour which may be due to increased adrenal activity caused by the remedy (Abramova *et al.*, 1972).

Siberian ginseng has also been shown in laboratory studies to combat the effects of radiation and chemical carcinogens and increase resistance to certain bacterial and fungal infections including *Candida albicans.*

In general, Siberian ginseng is ideal to take whenever extra energy is needed – before a particularly busy period at work, during exams or before long-distance air travel, for example. For longer-term use the usual recommendation is to use the herb for six weeks followed by a two week break. Like other potent tonic herbs it is best saved for those times when it is really needed rather than simply as a long-term supplement to combat an inadequate lifestyle.

It can help reduce the effects of jet lag and is an ideal all-round energy tonic, considered to be rather gentler than Korean ginseng and more suitable for women.

REISHI MUSHROOM

Botanical name: Ganoderma lucidem

Part used: fruiting body

How to use: capsules/powder – up to 1g daily

Use of this red bracket fungus – known in China as *Ling Zhi* – dates back to the days of the early emperors. The plant is now better known in the West by its Japanese name of *reishi* mushroom. *Ling Zhi* was highly regarded by the ancient Taoists as a spiritual tonic and one which could enhance longevity by helping to strengthen the disciple's determination to follow the path of virtue, central to Taoist belief.

On a physical level, the fungus has been shown to stimulate the immune system, lower blood sugar and cholesterol levels; it is also a sedative and an expectorant. It contains a number of polysaccharides which have potent anti-tumour properties and will lower blood pressure and act as a heart tonic (Willard,1990). It has been recommended in AIDS therapy and is used in Asia for degenerative diseases associated with ageing such as chronic bronchitis, coronary heart disease, high blood pressure and cancer.

Reishi, like many mushrooms, is known to contain complex sugars or polysaccharides which will stimulate the immune system and counter tumours. These are mainly types of glucan and ganoderan; there are also several triterpenes which are similar chemicals to those often found in aromatic essential oils. These include ganodermic acid and ganodermadiol and have been shown to reduce raised blood pressure and cholesterol levels as well as provide some protection for the liver against toxins. The mushroom also contains a steroid-like compound (ganodosterone) and an alkaloid which is believed to act as a heart tonic.

Reishi was once only gathered from the wild and was rare and very expensive. However, commercial cultivation began in Japan in the 1970s and the fungus is now widely grown on specially treated plum tree sawdust. Kits for growing *reishi* at home are also available. Commercial cultivation has brought a wide range of *reishi* capsules, powders and tinctures on to the heath food shop shelves. The usual dose is up to 1g daily.

Reishi is ideal as a calming sedative for anxiety, insomnia and nervousness as well as a useful tonic for debility and exhaustion. Following original Taoist use, it can also be regarded as a tool for strengthening our own will to make the necessary changes in lifestyle and habits that will lead to a healthier way of life.

Cautions: haemophiliacs are generally advised to avoid *reishi* although research studies have shown conflicting results.

KOREAN GINSENG

Botanical name: Panax ginseng

Part used: root

How to use: capsules – usually 600mg daily; tincture – up to 5ml, three times daily.

Ginseng has been regarded as something of a 'wonder drug' for at least 5,000 years. Originating in China, where it has long been used to strengthen the vital energy (*Qi*) of the body, the herb was known to Arab physicians by the ninth century, mentioned by Marco Polo in the thirteenth and introduced into modern Europe in the seventeenth century when a delegation from the King of Siam visited Louis XIV at Versailles and presented him with a root of 'gintz-æn'.

Ginseng has always been an expensive and highly prized herb that had, ideally, to be gathered in the wild using roots that were several years old. Today all ginseng is cultivated and it is an important cash crop.

The Chinese believe it is best suited to the elderly, preferring other energy tonics for those under forty, while many herbalists regard it as more suitable for men than women since it raises *yang* energy. The Chinese also believe it acts on the lungs and spleen and so can be helpful during recovery from chest problems – such as asthma – and digestive disorders.

Ginseng has been extensively researched in recent years and is known to contain a complex mixture of steroidal saponins which are believed to be primarily responsible for its action. Several of these compounds are very similar to human sex hormones – hence ginseng's reputation as an aphrodisiac. One recent study (Hong *et al.*, 2002) found that ginseng, at a dosage of 900mg, three times daily, had a significant effect on men suffering from erectile dysfunction. Some 60 per cent of the patients given Korean ginseng reported improved erection.

Like Siberian ginseng, the Korean species is termed an 'adaptogen' helping the body to adapt to stressful situations. During prolonged periods of tension it has been shown to reduce production of glucocorticoids by the adrenal cortex so helping to ameliorate the 'flight or fight' effect of stressful stimulation (Hiai *et al.*, 1979).

Like its Siberian cousin, ginseng has also been shown in clinical trials to enhance stamina and improve performance – although the experimental results have been rather more mixed. It seems to be most effective with male subjects – as one might expect from a strongly *yang* tonic. Researchers (Dorling *et al.*, 1980) found that about 1g of root given for twelve weeks produced a significant improvement in performance in simple physical tests. The same researchers subsequently ran a series of trials involving athletes and varying ginseng doses with similar improvements in performance but no quantifiable difference in improvement if the ginseng dose was doubled. The effect is not long term., however, and diminished rapidly once medication had ceased.

Korean ginseng is also known to stimulate the immune system and shows some anti-cancer activity. In a widespread study in South Korea, where ginseng is almost as commonly offered as a beverage as tea or coffee, researchers have concluded that the relative risk of cancer for ginseng users was half that of the non-drinkers (Yun and Choi, 1995).

As a general tonic it is ideally taken for a month in late autumn when the weather is changing from hot summer to cold winter and the body needs to adapt to the new environment, although the herb can, of course, be taken whenever there are problems due to tiredness and overwork. Ginseng will also reduce blood sugar and cholesterol levels and helps to stimulate the immune system.

Cautions: ginseng is best avoided in pregnancy although it may be taken then in small quantities for short periods. Other herbal stimulants, such as caffeine-containing drinks and horseradish – should be avoided while taking ginseng.

AMERICAN GINSENG

Botanical name: Panax quinquefolius

Parts used: root

How to use: capsules – usually 600mg daily; tincture – up to 5ml, three times daily

American ginseng was 'discovered' by Jesuit priests in Canada in the early eighteenth century, by 1765 it had entered the Chinese *Materia Medica* and by the 1787 legendary backwoodsmen, like Daniel Boone, were trading tonnes of the roots, making more profit from herbal medicine than from the fur trade.

The herb was largely used by Native Americans to ease stomach cramps and menstrual pains and as a tonic. The Menoni and Cherokee both called the plant 'little man' and the herb was regularly given to any wounded in battle as a supportive tonic to speed recovery.

In China – where the herb is known as *Xi Yang Shen* literally meaning 'root from the western seas' – it was regarded as a gentler, more *yin* remedy than the native Korean ginseng. It is mainly used to nourish *Qi*, fluids and lung *yin.* It is used in China for chronic coughs associated with lung deficiency (as in tuberculosis) and with low-grade fevers.

Recent laboratory studies (Duda *et al.*, 1999) have shown that the herb can also inhibit the growth of certain types of breast cancer cells and seems also to enhance the effect of more conventional drugs, such as tamoxifen. Other researchers have focused on the effect American ginseng has on blood sugar levels (Vuksan *et al.*, 2000) in sufferers of late-onset diabetes.

In general, American ginseng makes a gentle energy tonic for fatigue and debility in chronic disorders and convalescence when a stronger *yang* tonic would be inappropriate.

GUARANA

Botanical name: Paullinia cupana

Parts used: seeds

How to use: capsules – up to 2g daily

Guarana has been known in the West as an energy-elixir since the seventeenth century when missionaries reported that members of the Maués-Saterés tribe used the seeds as currency (much as the Aztecs did with cocoa beans) and carried them on journeys to take for hunger, fatigue, fevers, headaches and muscle cramps. The seeds, used medicinally, are found in bunches like red grapes on this rainforest shrub. The plant was originally a climber but centuries of cultivation have produced a shrubby form which is widely grown today.

It is a popular everyday drink in Brazil – much preferred to coffee – and is believed to stimulate the nervous system, improve concentration, and speed recovery after illness. It is also used to encourage urination in cystitis and other urinary tract disorders, as a painkiller for menstrual problems, and to relieve the discomfort of extreme heat.

Guarana contains a caffeine-like compound called guaranine, which is slower to metabolise so gives a gentler, more sustained stimulating effect than the artificial high of strong coffee.

The herb is usually promoted in the West as an energy-giving tonic. It can be helpful in chronic fatigue syndrome and is sometimes suggested for seasonal affective disorder (SAD) – a condition characterised by tiredness and depression in the winter months (van Straten, 1994).

Caution: avoid in high blood pressure and heart disease.

GOLDEN ROOT

Botanical name: Rhodiola rosea

Part used: root

How to use: 5–10 drops of tincture up to three times a day before meals

Golden root or rose root is a member of the Crassulaceae growing in dry sandy soils at high altitudes in the Arctic regions of Europe and Asia. It has been used for centuries in folk medicine in Russia and Scandinavia for a wide range of ailments including colds, influenza, impotence, cancers, anaemia and depression.

As with other traditional energy tonics the roots were regularly chewed to stave off hunger and fatigue and also to increase stamina: the Vikings reputedly used the herb to increase strength and endurance (Brown *et al.*, 2002).

Golden root appeared in the first Swedish *Pharmacopoeia* published in 1755 and has been extensively studied by Northern European researchers ever since. The plant is known to come into the adaptogen category capable of providing protection for stress, toxins and cold. A large number of active constituents have been identified, including phenylpropanoids, flavanoids, terpenes and phenolic acids which are generallly believed to account for its actions.

The herb is now largely regarded as an anti-fatigue remedy in small doses although larger amounts tend to have a more sedating effect. It stimulates production of several neurotransmitters and in animal studies has been found to improve learning abilities and memory (see Brown *et al.*, 2002 for an extensive literature review). Clinical trials have also confirmed this action with large-scale studies confirming that the herb can reduce fatigue, irritability, headaches, muscle weakness and general lack of energy. One Swedish study (Spasov *et al.*, 2000) used a standardised extract containing 3 per cent rosavin and 0.8 per cent salidroside (respectively, two of golden root's phenylpropanoid and phenylethanol constituents) giving a very low dose, which nevertheless produced significant improvements in physical fitness, well-being, and final exam grades for the students taking the remedy. Other researchers have reported improvements in depressed and psychotic patients taking similar low doses of golden root, while other trials (see Brown *et al.*, 2002) have found significant improvement in physical performance among Olympic athletes using the herb.

As well as reducing fatigue and improving stamina and performance golden root has also been shown to protect the heart especially during times of emotional and physical stress, helping to balance hormone production and nervous activity to normalise the system.

As a result of these various studies, golden root has become increasingly popular as an over-the-counter remedy; so much so that several species of *Rhodiola* are being marketed – although researchers suggest that it is only *R. rosea* which displays the full range of energising and anti-stress activity. The herb is also under investigation for use in Parkinson's disease, infertility and menstrual disorders, sexual dysfunction and chronic fatigue syndrome.

Caution: golden root can interfere with sleep patterns so is best taken early in the day; it should be avoided in manic-depressive syndromes.

ROSEMARY

Botanical name: Rosmarinus officinalis

Parts used: leaves, essential oil

How to use: infusion – 25g of fresh rosemary leaves to 500ml of boiling water, taken in three equal doses; tincture – up to 4ml/80 drops, three times a day' essential oil – 10 drops to 5ml of almond oil as a massage for aches and pains

Rosemary is traditionally associated with remembrance – sprigs were exchanged by lovers or scattered on coffins. It is an apt association as rosemary has a stimulating effect on the nervous system and a reputation for improving the memory. The plant originates from the Mediterranean area and was first grown in Britain in the fourteenth century. It was regarded as uplifting and energising – or as Gerard said, 'It comforteth the harte and maketh it merie'.

As a nerve tonic it can be helpful for temporary fatigue and overwork: take rosemary tea to relieve headaches, migraines, mild depression and coldness associated with poor circulation. It is a pleasant-tasting drink and, since rosemary is an evergreen, one that can be made using fresh herb throughout the year. The herb is also a good digestive remedy, helping to stimulate bile flow and improve function as well as clearing gas from the digestive tract. It will also increase urination and has some antiseptic properties, so that it makes a pleasant tasting addition to teas for ailments such as cystitis.

The essential oil made by steam-distilling the leaves is a valuable remedy for arthritis, rheumatism and muscular aches and pains. Rosemary is also traditionally used to darken hair colour and restore colour to grey hair as well as combating dandruff: add a few drops of oil or a cup of rosemary infusion to rinsing water after shampooing to help clear dandruff and improve the hair quality.

Studies in recent years (*Herbs for Health*, 1998; Svoboda and Deans 1990) have also confirmed that rosemary is a highly effective anti-oxidant which means that it can help to prevent cell decay and damage. It has been used in experimental treatments for Alzheimer's disease and, while not representing a cure, can help to slow the progression of the illness and help combat further decline.

Caution: avoid high doses of rosemary and use of rosemary oil in pregnancy.

DAMIANA

Botanical name: Turnera diffusa var. *aphrodisiaca*

Parts used: leaves

How to use: tincture – up to 3ml/60 drops, per dose, three times a day; infusion – 20 g to 500ml water taken in three equal doses; capsules up to 600 g daily

Damiana is a popular stimulant and aphrodisiac used to combat fatigue and give energy. It is an aromatic shrub found largely in Central and South America and acts as a restorative tonic for the nervous system. The leaves are used as a substitute for tea in Mexico and the plant is also used to flavour various South American liqueurs.

The plant has been poorly researched and although it is a popular nerve tonic and appears to strengthen male hormones there is very little understanding of its action or constituents. Damiana has long been used for impotence, loss of libido and premature ejaculation but it is also a strengthening tonic for the female reproductive system and is often given for painful or delayed periods.

It can be helpful in convalescence and general debility, both as a tonic and to encourage the appetite, and the herb is also mildly anti-depressant: it is generally labelled as 'thymoleptic' which means 'mood enhancing' – positively uplifting. Damiana is also a urinary antiseptic and will encourage urination so can be used for treating conditions like cystitis and other urinary tract problems.

Damiana is thus a valuable remedy for combating depression with a positive effect on mood. It is not a sedative, but as a restorative can be helpful if nervous exhaustion is at the root of the problem.

It is often combined with saw palmetto for male sexual problems, with oats and vervain for depression, or with raspberry leaf and St John's wort for menstrual discomfort and irregularity.

ASHWAGHANDA

Botanical name: Withania somnifera

Parts used: root, leaves, seed

How to use: powder – up to 5g in warm milk twice daily; tincture – up to 5ml per dose, three times a day

Known in English as winter cherry, *Withania somnifera* is becoming more familiar under its Sanskrit name, *ashwaghanda*, which translates as 'that which has the smell of a horse' as the plant was believed to endow any who took it with the strength, vitality and sexual energy of a horse.

It is one of Ayurvedic medicine's most important tonic herbs and has been studied extensively in recent years showing significant anti-tumour activity in laboratory tests. The herb is sometimes called 'Indian ginseng'; it is currently much less expensive than Korean ginseng and can be just as effective.

Unlike ginseng, which can be a very aggressive, overstimulating herb, *ashwaghanda* has a more sedating action so is a good restorative and soothing remedy where nervous exhaustion and stress are affecting behaviour and performance. It is often described as 'adaptogenic' which means that it helps the body to adapt to strains and stresses by stimulating our own defence mechanisms. As such it is far less invasive than pharmaceutical drugs which effectively 'take over' natural processes; instead adaptogenics work with, rather than against, natural functions.

Ashwaghanda is known to contain a number of potent alkaloids and saponins called sitoindosides, as well as chemicals called steroidal lactones (the withanolides and withaferins). These have been shown to be anti-bacterial, anti-tumour, and anti-inflammatory. They also behave rather like the glucocortocoid hormones produced in the body to enhance management of glucagon which is responsible for the release of sugars stored in the liver. The alkaloids have been shown to have a sedative effect while the sitoindosides have been shown to give some protection against stress-related disorders as well as improve the memory and learning ability in laboratory animals (Bone,1996).

As a traditional remedy in India, *ashwaghanda* is believed to encourage healthy growth in children and to combat emaciation caused by famine. This body-building capability was confirmed in the 1980s in a double-blind trial which involved giving *ashwaghanda* in milk to fifty-eight normal children. All those taking the fortified milk gained in body weight and plasma proteins and a strengthened hand-grip (Venkatraghava *et al.*, 1980).

Ashwaghanda can also increase vigour and energy in the elderly and – in one clinical trial – improved sexual performance in more than 70 per cent of the over-fifties men involved (Kuppurajan *et al.*, 1980). Studies have also shown that as well as helping to increase body weight, the herb slows the development of lung cancers in laboratory animals, and combats iron-deficient anaemia.

Although the root is mainly used, the leaves are taken in India in teas to encourage sleep in exhaustion and fevers, while the seeds have been shown to help protect against aspirin- and stress-induced ulcers, although they are traditionally avoided in Ayurvedic medicine as toxic (Bone, 1996).

Ashwaghanda can be a useful remedy for stress-related problems: it shows some sedative and soporific activity and has a traditional reputation for nurturing the mind and clarifying mental awareness. The traditional dose is 5g of powder twice a day in warm water sweetened with sugar and – so far – there seem to be no adverse reports of toxic effects in long-term use.

Mostly uplifting

Earlier herbals commonly remind us just how uplifting herbs can be: that particular plants will 'lift the spirits' or 'maketh the hart merrie'. The seventeenth century essayist John Evelyn describes lemon balm as 'powerfully chasing away melancholy', Nicholas Culpeper suggests of motherwort that 'there is no better herb to take melancholy vapours from the heart and make a merry, cheerful and lithe spirit', while John Gerard reminds us that roses are 'refreshing for the spirit'.

Many traditionally uplifting plants – notably lemon balm and St John's wort – are now known to be effective anti-depressants and have become very popular, especially with German physicians, as an alternative to pharmaceutical drugs. Their action tends to be slower and gentler so they may need to be taken for longer before producing the desired effect but many also have the benefit of fewer side-effects.

OATS

Botanical name: Avena sativa

Parts used: seeds, unripe aerial parts

How to use: juice – 10ml, three times a day; tincture – up to 5ml, three times a day. Porridge – add one cup of medium oatmeal to 1 litre of a 65:35 mixture of milk and water, add a pinch of salt and leave overnight in a well-buttered dish in a slow cooker or the simmering oven of an Aga

Oats – despite Dr Johnson's dismissal as 'a grain which in England is generally given to horses, but in Scotland supports the people' – are one of the world's most important cereal crops, used as a staple food in northern Europe for centuries. Oats are sweet, nutritious and warming – ideal to combat a cold, damp, northern climate. They are rich in iron, zinc and manganese, so are also a good source of many vital minerals.

Oatstraw, grains, bran and fresh whole plant are all used medicinally in various ways. The oatstraw and grains are especially anti-depressant and make a good restorative nerve tonic which is regarded as emotionally uplifting, so a bowl of porridge made from good-quality oatmeal is the ideal way to start the day. According to Weiss (1988) there have also been studies on traditional British night-time drinks of oats, barley and milk which have demonstrated that those drinking them before bed had a quieter, more restful night's sleep than control subjects who did not. This was especially true for older subjects.

Oatstraw tincture is generally used in herbal medicine and is often combined with vervain for nervous problems, exhaustion and depression, emotional upsets associated with the menopause, or debility following illness. The juice of fresh oats, pressed when still green, is similarly used as a nerve tonic.

Studies by Anand (1971), based on the use of oats to combat opium addiction in Ayurvedic medicine, found that the plant was also helpful in combating nicotine withdrawal symptoms among heavy smokers. Taking oat extracts helped reduce the number of cigarettes smoked and the effect persisted for two months after the end of the treatment. Oats act as a sedative so heavy smokers, who use cigarettes as an aid for relaxation, actually needed to smoke less frequently.

Oatstraw baths are used in folk medicine to counter rheumatic pains and the fresh plant is also used in homoeopathy for rheumatism. As a home remedy oatmeal is excellent in skin washes for eczema and dry skin – add a tablespoon to a bowl of warm water and use for washing. Writing in 1597, John Gerard certainly considered it as a beauty aid at a time when white skin was highly regarded: 'Oatmeale is good for to make a faire and well coloured maide,' he wrote, 'to looke like a cake of tallow'.

Recent research suggests that oatbran (and to a lesser extent oatmeal) can also help to reduce blood cholesterol levels, so it should certainly be included in the diet of those at risk from heart disease or atherosclerosis.

Oats can certainly be relaxant and sedative to relieve anxiety and insomnia – but do they also have an effect on mood? The late Hein Zeylstra FNIMH, who for many years ran the UK's School of Phytotherapy in Sussex, always used to cite the behaviour of race horses fed on oats to suggest that it might: such horses, he used to say, were always bright, alert and eager adding that 'you never see a miserable race horse'. Studies are lacking, but perhaps oats really do make us feel more alert and cheerful.

BORAGE

Botanical name: Borago officinalis

Parts used: leaves, seed oil

How to use: leaf infusion – 25g to 500 ml boiling water taken in three doses; tincture- up to 5ml three times daily; juice – 10ml, three times daily; seed oil capsules – typically 500mg per day

The old country saying 'borage for courage' is a rather apt description of the plant since we now know that it will stimulate production of the hormone adrenaline – the 'flight or fight' hormone which we produce in moments of stress. Borage has also long been regarded as uplifting for the emotions. It has been identified with the Roman *euphrosynum*, 'the plant that cheers', which Pliny tells us was once added to wine to 'increase the exhilarating effect', while Elizabethan cooks added blue borage flowers to salads to 'make the mind glad': borage flowers are still traditionally added to summer drinks like Pimms.

The herb is also soothing for irritant tissues and generally regarded as mildly sedative and anti-depressant although there has been little research into these properties.

In recent years borage has come to the fore as a rich source of *gamma*-linolenic acid (GLA) an essential fatty acid which is found in the pressed seed oil. Like evening primrose oil, borage has thus become a favourite with the health food industry. GLA, is needed by the body for a number of metabolic processes and lack of it can be associated with menstrual irregularities, skin problems, irritable bowel syndrome and rheumatoid arthritis.

Borage oil is often sold as 'starflower oil' – this is not a traditional name, but one which probably appeals to the marketeers. It contains substantially more GLA than evening primrose oil, with around 24 per cent (compared with a figure of 9 per cent generally quoted for evening primrose). However, traces of toxic erucic acid (which is known to damage heart tissue) are sometimes found in the oil, leading to claims that evening primrose oil is more efficacious.

Borage is also related to comfrey and traces of chemicals called pyrrolizidine alkaloids – which, in large quantities, can cause liver damage – have been found in its leaves. It has therefore been banned in some countries, although most herbalists regard it as perfectly safe for regular use. The leaves can be used in teas for stress or to counter the lingering effects of steroid therapy and they can also be added to cough mixtures to help clear phlegm. The juice can be used internally as a natural anti-depressant to improve well-being while externally it makes a soothing lotion for irritant skin rashes and inflammations.

BALMONY

Botanical name: Chelone glabra

Parts used: aerial parts

How to use: 25g dried leaf to 500ml of boiling water for infusions; 20 drops of tincture per dose

Balmony is another poorly researched plant. Originating in North America, it thrives in wet woodland and marshy areas. It is known as turtlebloom in the USA – the flower head is said to resemble a turtle and *chelone* is derived from the Greek word for tortoise. The herb was traditionally used to clear intestinal worms and as a digestive and appetite stimulant in debility and constipation. In the nineteenth century it came to be regarded as an anti-depressant by the eclectics – a US herbal movement which also became popular in the UK – and is used as such by many traditional western herbalists today.

It is primarily a liver stimulant and tonic which can be helpful in gall bladder problems, colic and jaundice but is often added to anti-depressant mixtures. Many liver stimulants were traditionally used in Galenic medicine to clear excess yellow and black bile which were believed to cause, respectively, bad temper and melancholy.

BLACK COHOSH

Botanical name: Cimicifuga racemosa

Parts used: rhizome

How to use: up to 2ml of tincture or 200mg in capsules daily.

Black cohosh is a traditional North American plant. which arrived in Europe in the nineteenth century. It was very widely used by Native Americans for yellow fever, colic, 'hysterical affections', snakebite, sore throats, and kidney problems, as well as for an impressive list of gynaecological problems. It was regarded as a key remedy for rheumatism and as such it was a 'favourite remedy' of the nineteenth century American eclectic physician John King (1813–93), who used it for both acute and chronic cases of rheumatism and for other inflammatory conditions including respiratory problems and neuralgia (Foster, 1999).

The herb is also sedative and relaxing and as a traditional remedy for hysterical states and melancholy.

Studies during the 1950s and 1960s identified its main constituents as various triterpene glycosides including xyloside and cimicifugoside as well as possibly isoflavone, but much of this research has produced conflicting results and little is really known of its active principles.

Recent studies have focused on its gynaecological action and several (detailed in Foster, 1999) have confirmed that it effectively relieves menopausal symptoms. It is particularly appropriate for depression or emotional lability associated with the menopause.

Researchers currently disagree as to its actual action with some suggesting that it has oestrogenic-like activity while others maintain that it is non-hormonal. Whatever its action, the herb has been shown in trials to relieve all sorts of menopausal discomforts including hot flushes, sweating, and sleep disturbances, as well as nervous problems. It is now a very popular over-the-counter remedy for menopausal problems, although it can also be helpful for breast discomfort associated with premenstrual syndrome. Traditionally the herb was used to prevent threatened miscarriage, although such use requires skill and experience and is not an area for home remedies.

Black cohosh is also still popular for aches and pains and is included in many over-the-counter remedies for arthritis and rheumatism: it is recommended for cramps, sciatica, back pain, facial neuralgia and aches and pains following strenuous exercise.

Cautions: excess can cause nausea and vomiting and the herb should be avoided in pregnancy.

LADY'S SLIPPER

Botanical name: Cypredium pubescens

Parts used: root

How to use: 15–20g to 750ml of water as a decoction taken in three doses; up 40–60 drops of tincture, three times daily

This beautiful North American orchid was widely used as a sedative, relaxant, painkiller and thymoleptic to combat a variety of nervous problems ranging from insomnia and anxiety through to depression and schizophrenia.

The plant was once a popular home remedy in North America and was considered as especially suitable for women and children: it was used to ease painful menstruation and in labour and was popular for sleepless and restless children. The plant proved so popular that it is now seriously endangered and its medicinal use should be severely restricted. There is some limited cultivation, but orchids are never easy to grow in artificial environments. Wild harvested supplies should definitely be avoided.

Both the yellow lady's slipper orchid (*C. pubescens*) and the pink form (*C. acaule*) were used by Native Americans – the Menominees preferred the yellow as a remedy for women and the pink for men (Vogel, 1960).

The herb is very poorly researched but throughout the nineteenth and much of the twentieth centuries it was widely and effectively used for a range of nervous problems including hysteria, depression, nervous headaches and insomnia. It is an effective tranquilliser with a restorative action creating a very positive and uplifting remedy which is now sadly so rarely available.

GINKGO

Botanical name: Ginkgo biloba

Parts used: leaves, seeds

How to use: tincture (leaf) – up to 15ml daily; capsules (leaf) – up to 2g daily

Ginkgo is something of a botanical anachronism – a rare, prehistoric deciduous conifer, unchanged since before the evolution of mammals. It owes its survival to preservation as a sacred plant in temple gardens in China and Japan and was introduced into Europe in 1727 when it became popular as a botanical garden ornamental. Some of Europe's oldest ginkgo trees – also known as maidenhair trees – can be found in the Chelsea Physic Garden in London and the Jardin des Plantes in Paris.

Although the Chinese have prescribed the seeds (known as *Bai Guo*) for asthma and urinary problems for many centuries, it is only in the past few years that the herb has been used medicinally in the West. Research in the past decade has highlighted its action as a platelet-activating factor (PAF) which counters the allergic response – reinforcing its traditional use as an anti-asthmatic (Lane and Fauci, 1985). More significantly, ginkgo leaf extracts have been shown to improve cerebral circulation. In laboratory tests the herb has been shown to prevent the damage which can be caused by restricted blood flow – as in strokes – and there are also suggestions that it can prevent nerve damage also caused by restricted blood flow (Mills and Bone, 2000). It can be especially helpful for depression in the elderly which can be associated with the type of confusion caused by this restriction in blood supply to the brain. In Germany it has been tested on patients after brain surgery following strokes, and been found to improve recovery rates dramatically (Maier-Hauff, 1992).

Its action in strengthening the cerebral circulation has led many to regard it as an anti-ageing remedy, since hardening of the arteries in the brain is a common cause of apparent confusion in the elderly. It is generally beneficial for many circulatory ailments (including, according to some researchers, varicose veins) and its effect on cerebral circulation has also led to its use in the treatment of Ménières disease and tinnitus.

Adding to its use as an anti-ageing remedy, is ginkgo's anti-oxidant activity. Flavonoids from the herb have been shown to scavenge the free radicals which can cause cell damage (Joyeux *et al.*, 1995). Ginkgo extract was also found to reduce signs of oxidative damage in the blood of salvage workers involved in clearance after the Chernobyl nuclear accident (Emerit *et al.*, 1995). The workers were given 120mg a day of a standardised ginkgo extract for two months after which time their blood plasma had returned to normal.

Other researchers have focused on ginkgo's reputation for improving memory and learning with a number of well-controlled studies showing that ginkgo can have a positive effect on learning skills. In short-term trials involving very high doses of ginkgo there was an impressive improvement in cognitive function (Subhan and Hindmarch, 1986) although the researchers suggest that lower doses over a longer time period could have a similar effect.

Numerous other studies have focused on ginkgo's effectiveness at reducing tinnitus and combating hearing loss, reducing symptoms of vertigo, generally improving cerebral circulation, reducing the effects of arterial diseases and helping with various eye disorders linked to poor circulation or blocked veins (see Mills and Bone, 2000 for review). The herb has also shown efficacy in treating Alzheimer's-type senile dementia. In one study, patients were given 240mg of ginkgo extract daily and after one month memory and attention span had improved significantly (Hofferberth, 1994). A more recent project (Solomon, 2002) looked at memory enhancement in a group of healthy elderly patients. It found no significant difference between the ginkgo regime or placebo confirming that the herb is really only helpful where there is an inherent pathological problem.

Much of the research has focused on standardised ginkgo extracts, rather than the crude herb which has been poorly researched. The German Commission E monograph, widely regarded as a comprehensive guide to the plants safety and uses, recommends the standardised extract for symptoms of dementia – including poor concentration, headache, dizziness and tinnitus – as well as vertigo and tinnitus related to circulatory disorders, and problems linked to peripheral arterial disorders.

Crude ginkgo is widely sold as a food supplement and can be usefully taken by the elderly or those with chronic circulatory disorders, although in the UK standardised extracts are less commonly available over-the-counter.

ST JOHN'S WORT

Botanical name: Hypericum perforatum

Parts used: flowering tops, leaves

How to use: tincture – 4ml/80 drops up to three times daily; capsules – up to 250mg, three times daily; infusion – 25g to 500ml water taken in three equal doses

Although a traditional wound herb and pain remedy, St John's wort is now better known as an anti-depressant. In Germany it is one of the more popular remedies prescribed by orthodox physicians and as such it has had its share of bad publicity and widely reported adverse side-effects,

The plant is believed to take its name from the Knights of St John of Jerusalem who used it as a wound herb on Crusade battlefields – although others suggest that it is associated with the midsummer rites of St John's Day (24 June) and the blood-red extracts that can be obtained from the herb. It is a good example of the Doctrine of Signatures, which reasoned that the appearance of plants contained clues as to their use to guide mere mortals to select the right remedy. St John's wort's red extracts implied blood and inflammation so the plant was used to treat these sorts of traumatic injuries. It is, in fact, a very effective antiseptic and anti-inflammatory when used externally: useful in home first aid for grazes and minor burns. The plant produces bright yellow flowers in early to midsummer and these can be collected and infused in sunflower oil for two weeks to produce a red oil which is ideal for soothing minor burns and sunburn.

St John's wort was believed to ward off evil spirits and the insane were often compelled to drink an infusion in an attempt to cure their madness. Today we know that the herb is an effective anti-depressant which is believed to inhibit the enzyme monoamine oxidase (MAO), which itself inhibits neurotransmitters involved in stimulating the brain. MAO inhibitors are widely used in orthodox medicine and some researchers suggest St John's wort has a similar action.

The herb has been successfully used in seasonal affective disorder (SAD), for emotional upsets associated with the menopause, and for mild cases of depression. St John's wort has long been regarded by herbalists as a restorative for the nervous system and it can ease pre-menstrual tension and some types of period pain. Research in recent years has also focused on its action as an immune system and the herb has been used in AIDS treatments (Cooper and James, 1990).

Over the past two decades, there have been numerous clinical trials examining the anti-depressant activity of St John's wort. The herb's efficacy has been compared with various conventional anti-depressant drugs such as fluoxetine (a selective serotonin re-uptake inhibitor) and imipramine, one of the tricyclic antidepressants (Broughton, 1999). Results have tended to be positive with St John's wort performing as well as the orthodox remedies and generally with fewer reported side-effects. However, not all researchers agree that hypericin is really the component responsible for St John's wort's anti-depressant action and other chemicals – such as hyperforin which acts rather like fluoxetine – should be investigated.

A review of twenty-three clinical trials (Linde *et al.*, 1996) involving 1757 depressed patients confirmed that St John's wort extract was more effective than a placebo in both mild and moderately severe cases.

Many of these trials have involved standardised extracts of St John's wort containing a known amount of hypericin, one of its constituents; dosages tend to be quite high at around 5g of herb extract daily. This emphasis on concentrated extracts has also led to major concerns over the safety of the herb. In 1999 newspaper reports began to quote US warnings that high and prolonged doses of St John's wort could trigger cataracts in people who were subsequently exposed to bright lights (*Daily Telegraph,* 22 July 1999) warning that this could be significant for those using the herb to treat seasonal affective disorder (SAD) where therapy can often involve exposure to prolonged artificial daylight.

By early 2000, reports of liver damage associated with taking high doses of hypericin extracts in conjunction with other drugs were starting to appear (Ernst, 2000). In the same year the Irish Medicines Board made St John's wort a prescription-only drug and in the UK the Department of Health and Medicines Control Agency issued new guidelines warning that St John's wort could interact with numerous common drugs – from oral contraceptives to certain antibiotics – and urging professional herbalists to limit prescriptions.

Yet – as has happened with numerous other traditional herbal remedies in the past – the suspect medication in all this has not been whole plant extracts, as used by herbalists, but highly concentrated and standardised products often sold for self-medication and open to patient abuse. Equally, the sort of drug interactions that so worried the legislators involve a liver enzyme system called cytochrome P450 which is involved in the metabolism of many chemical compounds including some of those in both herbal and pharmaceutical drugs. However, liver drug metabolism varies enormously between individuals and is also affected by the foods we may have recently eaten so the evidence against St John's wort is at best flimsy (Broughton and Denham, 2000).

All the studies involving the herb and various drug interactions are based on a handful of cases and often there is very imprecise information about the patients' full drug regime. The Swedish health regulators, for example, reported problems with St John wort and oral contraceptives based on eight cases of intra-menstrual bleeding in women taking both medicines; three of the women recovered when they stopped taking St John's wort but the others were not followed up. Since intra-menstrual bleeding is a common problem with oral contraceptives it seems a little biased to damn the herb on such scanty evidence.

As Broughton and Denham also point out, all the adverse reactions involving St John's wort were the result of using standardised hypericin extracts. Caution is certainly recommended – as with any herb used in conjunction with powerful pharmaceutical drugs – but more detailed case studies of patients taking the whole plant extract in conjunction with other medication are needed before widespread restrictions are applied.

Used in moderation, St John's wort can be an effective sedative and relaxant to combat anxiety syndromes – although the fashion for standardised selective extracts could do more harm than good. Gather fresh herbs if available or use good quality whole dried plant material in infusions.

Cautions: excessively high doses and prolonged use have been linked to cataracts and nerve hypersensitivity; in rare cases prolonged use may increase the photosensitivity of the skin; current advice is to seek professional guidance before taking the herb if on prescription drugs.

YERBA MATÉ

Botanical name: Ilex paraguariensis

Parts used: dried leaves

How to use: 1–2 teaspoons per cup of boiling water, infused for 10 minutes as required

Maté is a national drink of Paraguay and Brazil, regarded as a good substitute for tea containing reasonably high levels of caffeine – around 1.5 per cent so less than guarana but more than coffee – as well as traces of theobromine.

The leaves are gathered when the berries are ripe, hung over a wood fire to dry and slightly roast, then powdered and stored for a year before the tea is used.

Like other herbs which are rich in caffeine, maté is stimulating and is used to give a short-term boost in energy levels. It stimulates the nervous system and – like similar plants can increase heart rate and act as a diuretic. It is good general tonic, ideal for physical exhaustion and stress-related problems, and is also widely drunk in parts of South America for mild depression.

It can be used instead of tea or coffee as an everyday drink to help support stronger herbal remedies in cases of nervous exhaustion and depression.

LEMON BALM

Botanical name: Melissa officinalis

Parts used: leaves, essential oil

How to use: infusion – 25g dried herb to 500ml boiling water taken in three equal doses daily; tincture – up to 6ml, three times daily

Lemon balm's botanical name, *Melissa,* comes from the Greek word *mel,* meaning honey, and the herb has a long association with bees and the healing power of their products. It is said to be such a favourite with bees that if hives are rubbed with its leaves the insects will never swarm and always return. Lemon balm was regarded by the Greeks as a cure-all and the herb has been considered over the centuries as being as valuable as honey for treating wounds and equal in tonic effect to royal jelly.

John Gerard declared that it '. . .comforteth the hart and driveth away all melancholie and sadnesse', while it was praised by the German herbalist Paracelsus as an 'elixir of youth' which he made into a preparation called *primum ens melissae*. As late as the eighteenth century lemon balm was still being recommended in 'canary wine' to 'renew youth'.

Lemon balm contains an essential oil which is rich in citral and citronellal; these have been shown to be calming for the nervous system. The oil is also rich in polyphenols, including rosmarinic acid, which are anti-viral and account for lemon balm's effectiveness in combating the *Herpes simplex* virus which is responsible for cold sores. This has been confirmed in a number of clinical trials involving more than 200 patients (ESCOP, 1996). The herb can be helpful for other viral infections, including mumps and shingles.

Today the plant is mainly used – much like chamomile – as a calming digestive remedy and sedative for treating nervous disorders; it is a gentle but potent herb ideal for nervous tummy upsets in children but also potent enough to help with depression and anxiety and to relieve tension headaches. It has been used successfully for quite severe conditions including post-natal depression.

ESCOP (1996) describes lemon balm as primarily suitable for 'tenseness, restlessness and irritability' as well as being applicable for digestive disorders. The monograph also adds that laboratory studies have demonstrated the herb's sedative action at low doses while at higher doses it is a more effective analgesic.

Lemon balm is also cooling and will encourage sweating so is useful to reduce body temperature in fevers. Modern research has shown it to be extremely effective against several bacteria and demonstrated that it can inhibit thyroid action, so that it can also be used to ease an over-active thyroid which may cause symptoms of anxiety.

Tea made from a handful of fresh leaves makes a refreshing and restorative drink at the end of the day. The herb needs to be dried with care to avoid losing too much of the characteristic lemon flavour due to evaporation of the citral and citronellal content. These degrade further with storage and some suggest that the plant is really only effective as a sedative when it is used either fresh or within six months of harvesting.

Externally, lemon balm creams can be used on insect bites, sores and slow-healing wounds. The essential oil is used in aromatherapy for nervous problems but is also valuable, well diluted in sprays, for keeping insects away.

Like chamomile, lemon balm is a convenient sedative remedy for anxiety; as Gerard noted, the rich lemon smell of the fresh herb is generally considered as uplifting and mood enhancing – it 'driveth away all sadnesse' – although there has been little formal investigation to confirm this sort of activity.

It is appropriate for anxiety and mild depression; is uplifting and contributes to any 'feel-good factor'.

BASIL

Botanical name: Ocimum spp.

Parts used: leaves, essential oil

How to use: fresh leaves – eat plenty in season or freeze for use in winter cooking; infusion – 25g of dried leaf to 500ml boiling water taken in three equal doses with a teaspoonful of honey; tincture – up to 4ml/80 drops three times a day; essential oil – add 5 drops to bath water or to 25ml of almond oil as a massage rub.

Familiar in Europe as a culinary herb *(O. basilicum)* sweet basil's close relative holy basil *(O. sanctum)* is regarded in India as a potent tonic – sacred to the deities Vishnu and Krishna, capable of 'opening the heart and mind', and second only to the lotus in a hierarchy of sacred plants. In Ayurveda it is believed to bestow love and devotion and is also used in chills to clear excess phlegm and catarrh (associated with the *kapha dosha*) from the nasal passages and lungs.

Although basil originates in India, the plant has been known in Europe since ancient times, although views and traditions associated with it have been mixed. The Greek physician Dioscorides said it should never be taken internally while the Roman Pliny recommended it for fainting, headaches, catarrh, indigestion and other digestive upsets, adding that as an aphrodisiac it was especially good for horses 'at the time of service'. He also added that many still believed that basil pounded in a mortar and left would 'breed a scorpion' if left covered by a stone or 'breed worms' if left in the sun. The Greeks and Romans also believed that the more you abused or scorned it the better it grew so planting the seeds was always accompanied with plenty of invective. In contrast, in parts of the Middle East it is still planted on graves in loving remembrance.

Today, basil is generally recommended in the West for digestive upsets and to clear intestinal parasites. It is important to remember its Eastern attributes and keep a basil plant in the house for its purifying and protective influence. In India basil is made into a tea with honey to promote clarity of mind while the stems are made into rosaries and worn to encourage clarity and compassion. The essential oil is popular in aromatherapy and can be used as a nerve tonic, anti-depressant and digestive remedy or be added to chest rubs for coughs and congestion. The fresh leaves can be useful topically for clear fungal infections on the skin.

Basil is worth considering for the mental clarity and positive moods it can encourage; the oil is a more potent nervine and anti-depressant, so add it to bath water to combat mild depression and eat plenty of fresh basil leaves with pasta and tomato dishes.

Caution: avoid basil oil in pregnancy.

ROSE

Botanical name: Rosa spp.

Parts used: petals, fruits, essential oil

How to use: R. damascena/R. centifolia: baths – 2 drops of rose oil to bath water for depression, sorrows or insomnia; massage oil: up to 10 drops of rose oil in 5ml of almond oil to relieve stress and exhaustion. *R. gallica:* tincture: up to 3ml, thrice daily for diarrhoea or sluggish digestion

There is a saying that roses are good for 'the skin and the soul' – or as *Askham's Herbal* put it in 1550 '. . .drye roses put to ye nose to smell do comforte the braine and the harte and quencheth sprite'.

Through the centuries roses have been used medicinally in all cultures for an enormous variety of ailments. In Roman times the wild rose (*R. canina*) was recommended – probably unsuccessfully – for the bites of rabid dogs. While in China the hips of the Cherokee rose (*R. laevigata*), known as *Jin Ying Zi*, are used mainly as a kidney *Qi* tonic also prescribed for urinary dysfunction. The hardy Japanese rose (*R. rugosa*), often used in hedging, is also used in Chinese medicine: the flowers (*Mei Gui Hua*) are regarded as a *Qi* stimulant and blood tonic to relieve stagnant liver energies. They are used for digestive irregularities or with motherwort for heavy periods. Roses continued as an official medicine in the UK well into the 1930s when tincture of apothecary's rose (*R. gallica*) was still dispensed by pharmacists for sore throats.

The plant was originally held sacred to Venus, but by the middle ages it had become symbolically associated with the Virgin Mary and the traditional Catholic rosary was once made of rolled rose leaves.

In ancient times roses were regarded as a panacea and the list of their reputed therapeutic properties is impressive. At various times they have been recommended for: hay fever, anxiety, diarrhoea, gall bladder problems, conjunctivitis, tonsillitis, excessive perspiration, poor circulation, vaginal thrush, *Herpes zoster*, *Herpes simplex*, constipation, depression, frigidity, haemorrhage, headache, liver congestion, impotence, insomnia, sleeplessness, heavy menstrual bleeding, nausea, nervous strain, eye pains, sterility, uterine diseases, vomiting and skin problems.

By the middle ages rose oil was the preferred remedy to treat the plague while Nicholas Culpeper writing in 1653 suggests a purgative rose syrup for constipation, rose water for various eye inflammations, and rose tincture for digestive and menstrual problems.

Most rose oil is collected from the damask rose (*R. damascena*). It can cost up to £7,500 a kilo and is one of the most important oils used in aromatherapy. Rose oil contains some 300 chemical constituents of which only around 100 have as yet been identified. According to German researcher Professor Dietrich Wabner (Ody,

1989) just nine of rose's constituents account for some 86 per cent of the oil's volume while the 190 or so still to be classified form only 1.4 per cent of the oil. These trace compounds give rose oil its distinctive fragrance and possibly much of its therapeutic value as well (Kovats, 1987). The most important trace element is called dehydro-*iso*-ionone, also known as *beta*-damascenone, and forms about 0.1 per cent of the oil. This is believed to be responsible for much of the potent honey fragrance of *R. damascena*.

Other known constituents (see Table 8) also have clearly defined therapeutic roles: citronellol, for example, is known as an insecticide and also has an anti-rheumatic effect; eugenol and phenyl ethanol are anaesthetic and anti-bacterial; farnesol is also anti-bacterial and has a beneficial effect on the skin; while citral is antiseptic. Phenyl ethanol also has a slightly narcotic effect and considerably more of this is present in French cabbage rose (*R. centifolia)* oil than in Bulgarian damask rose oil.

Unlike modern hybrid roses the damask rose blooms for only a couple of weeks when the petals are collected and steam distilled to produce true Bulgarian rose oil. The oil is used in around 96 per cent of all women's perfumes. Medicinally it is an important nervine used for depression and anxiety and can be helpful for those who lack love in their lives. On a physical level, it can be added to many skin remedies or used for digestive problems.

Roses are also highly astringent and so are recommended for

Table 8: Constituents found in Bulgarian rose otto and French rose absolute

	Bulgarian *R damascena*	French *R centifolia*
(-)- citronellol	34–55%	18–22%
phenyl ethanol	1.5–3%	*c.* 63%
geraniol and nerol	30–40%	10–15%
farnesol	0.2–2%	0.2–2%
stearopten	16–22%	*c.* 8%

There are also traces of nonalol, linalool, phenylacetaldehyde, citral, carvone, citronellyl acetate, 2–phenylmethyl acetate, methyl eugenol, and eugenol.

chronic diarrhoea, sore throats, severe cystitis and other ailments where drying excess secretions and soothing inflammations are important.

Roses are also important in the Ayurvedic medicine of India: *shatapatra* (*R. indica*) is generally considered cooling and a good tonic for the mind. The 'temperature' of rose preparations can be varied in Eastern tradition by leaving them in moonlight to cool the mixture or in sunshine to produce a more heating brew.

Roses are ideal to combat excessive anxiety (including panic attacks), stress and insomnia. The oil can best be used in baths, massage or as an inhalant (put 1–2 drops on a handkerchief and sniff frequently) while fresh petals can easily be made into a tincture at home and have a very soothing effect on the emotions when taken internally. Rose petal sandwiches and jams were Victorian delicacies well worth reviving for their therapeutic effects.

Rose also has a reputation for enhancing mental awareness while the list of its therapeutic actions though the ages is impressive. Roses in western society tend to be regarded as simply attractive flowers and love tokens; they are very under-rated as medicinal herbs and interest in them is overdue for a revival.

Cautions: because of the high price of rose oils adulteration is commonplace and only the best quality, genuine oils should be used medicinally.

VERVAIN

Botanical name: Verbena officinalis

Parts used: aerial parts.

How to use: tincture – up to 5ml, three times daily; infusion – 25g of dried herb to 500ml of boiling water taken in three equal doses daily

John Gerard – who clearly had little time for folk traditions – warns his readers not to listen to 'odde olde wives tales' of vervain that told of 'witchcraft and sorceries'. As late as the seventeenth century the plant was still being used in fortune-telling rites – a practice that can be traced back at least to Druidic times.

The Romans called it *hiera botane* (sacred plant) and used it to purify homes and spread on Jupiter's altars. Well into the Christian era it was castigated as a witch plant – or as the eleventh century writings of the physicians of Myddfai in Wales warn '. . .give no heed to those who say that it should be gathered in the name of the devil'. The Druids, according to Pliny, collected it when the 'dog star could be seen in the heavens'.

Medicinally it is used mainly as a relaxing remedy for nervous problems and as a liver tonic – bitter and stimulating for the digestion; it is an ideal tonic in convalescence and debility. Vervain can also be helpful for nerve pains and migraine – taken internally or applied topically in a compress. Vervain combines well with oats in depression and is a useful herb for nursing mothers – relaxing the nervous system to take the tension out of feeding time and stimulating milk flow.

Vervain is a good example of an holistic herb. It has a physical effect on the liver and nervous system. The Bach Flower Remedy based on vervain is recommended for 'tenseness, over-enthusiasm and over-effort' giving the plant an emotional dimension. On a spiritual level, some herbalists believe that it can heal holes in the human aura – the spiritual energy field, revealed by Kirlian photography, which is believed to surround each of us and indicate our inner well-being. Vervain is thus a very complete remedy which can ease anxiety and mild depression and can also have an effect on our emotional and spiritual well-being.

It is not well studied, although there have been some laboratory trials demonstrating its anti-tremor, analgesic and hypotensive properties (Newall *et al.*, 1996).

Caution: vervain should be avoided in pregnancy but can be taken in labour to stimulate contractions.

CHAPTER 5

Learning to relax

> You have to give up the pursuit of happiness in order to be happy. It is not outside us or somewhere in the future. We get stressed because we ought to be happier, and we are often waiting for it to happen. . . If you merely make a concrete choice to be happy, then you will become happier.
>
> Robert Holden, in *Happiness Now!*

While there are a great many herbal remedies for stress, anxiety, depression and insomnia, they can provide little long-term relief if the problems causing them are not also addressed. There may be issues of over-work, unhappy relationships or an over-extravagent lifestyle which need to be tackled.

Self-help manuals regularly tell us that we must 'learn to relax' – but that is a simple skill, one which is usually not too difficult to acquire and which has already spawned a thriving publishing industry. What is more important is to enjoy and be satisfied with whatever it is we are doing. If we can learn to cope with stress inputs, then we can avoid those negative stress responses which lead to so much ill health, and relaxation becomes a semi-permanent state – rather than something which must be contrived and worked at in between bouts of tense, unpleasant activity.

The fashionable gurus who quote the old Latin tag *carpe diem,* telling us to 'seize the day' and grab every opportunity that presents itself to us, should occasionally take a little time to remember the full quotation. It comes from Horace's *Odes: carpe diem, quam minimum credula postero* and is usually translated as 'enjoy today, trusting little to tomorrow' – a variant on 'make hay while the sun shines' or 'eat, drink and be merry, for tomorrow we die' – and reflects a rather more relaxed and hedonistic approach to life than the relentless activity and opportunism with which 'seize the day' is often imbued.

Setting achievable goals and priorities can ease many anxieties, as can simple techniques to encourage relaxation. Deep breathing exercises and some of the basic yoga or *Qigong* movements are easy to adopt and many of these simple exercises can be undertaken in odd moments of the day to ease tensions.

Qigong

Qigong is one of China's oldest exercise therapies and involves a combination of exercises and postures which focus the mind on the breath and energy flows through the body. Over the centuries techniques have evolved which encourage energy flows through the body's channels – the meridians used in acupuncture – and also stimulate blood circulation. Some of the routines are complex, ballet-like and beautiful, others can be quite simple and help to clear the mind and combat nervous tensions.

- *Simple standing* – this is believed to combat general tiredness and insomnia: stand upright, quite naturally, raising the crown of the head gently. With mouth closed, eyelids drooping and relaxed shoulders concentrate on a point below your navel. Serious students of *Qigong* will stand in this position for many hours concentrating totally on the energy centre below the navel and not permitting their minds to wander at all.
- *Sitting with hands facing* – this is a posture for developing more energy. Sit on the edge of a chair with a straight back, closed eyes and upright head. Put the tongue to the roof of the mouth and draw your feet back so that your toes are directly below the knees. Bend your arms at the elbow and raise your hands to

elbow height with the palms facing but not touching and concentrate on the space between the hands. If you feel a slight tingling sensation in your hands that is simply your *Qi* strengthening and flowing between the palms. Maintain the position for as long as your mind remains clear.

- *Releasing negative energy* – this is another sitting position which can help to relieve tension and tiredness. Sit on a chair as for the 'hands facing' posture, but this time with your feet in front of you and relax your ankles so that they turn over on their sides and rest with soles facing. Put your hands on your knees and focus on the energy flow at your feet for a few minutes.

T'ai-chi chuan

Sometimes classified as a martial art (*t'ai-chi chuan* is often called *t'ai-chi* boxing) the various *t'ai-chi* routines are designed to strengthen energy flows and were once used in a combative way – masters can 'throw their *Qi*' at opponents with enough power to knock them sideways. As well as stimulating body functions and healthy metabolism, *t'ai-chi* is believed to rebuild energy and clear the mind. As with *Qigong* the exercise routines involve precise breathing sequences and meditative concentration.

A typical *t'ai-chi* sequence can include 100 movements and it is usually taught gradually in classes, allowing students to learn the sequence and eventually practise the routine each day on their own. Once you know the exercise steps, it usually takes no more than 20 minutes to complete the entire cycle. Numerous books and videos are now available to teach *t'ai-chi*, although it is always better to start with a regular class and good teacher if possible.

Yoga

There are several yoga methods which focus predominantly either on the body – largely exercise and relaxation routines – or the spirit.

Hatha yoga is the most familiar and involves practising various postures or *asanas.* These usually involve holding a balancing or stretching pose for several minutes while concentrating on breath and focusing vital energy flows. *Hatha* teachers range from those who prefer the vigorous approach – such as followers of B. K. S. Iyengar's method – with lots of energetic jumping into positions, to others who take things at a more leisurely pace with plenty of lying on the floor relaxing in between postures. It is well worth checking on the approach of an individual teacher before signing up for classes.

In the non-physical yoga category come *karma* yoga – devotion to the service of others; *bhakti* yoga – devotion to the worship of God; and *jnana* yoga – an emphasis on learning and spiritual knowledge.

There are numerous postures in *hatha* yoga which can easily be incorporated into a relaxation regime, such as:

- *The tree pose* which involves standing on one leg with the other bent at the knee with the foot placed against the inner thigh. Once balance is secure raise the arms and place your hands, palms together, on the crown of the head. Repeat standing on the alternate leg; or
- *The locust* – lie on your tummy with the hands clenched and placed underneath the groin. Breath in and lift your legs from the hips with straight knees as high as possible at the same time pressing down with your hands. Hold for five seconds before lowering the legs and breathing out. Rest and repeat.

It is best to start yoga in classes with a good teacher and practise the postures for about twenty minutes each day. As in *Qigong,* yoga exercise always includes an element of breath control and it is also important to keep breathing synchronised to the various posture movements.

All the yogas also include an element of *rajah* yoga or meditation – usually based on a *mantra* or *mandala* – which also lays great stress on breathing exercises and control. Among the most popular breathing sequences are:

- Breathe in through your nose while counting up to five. Hold your breath for a further count of five and then breathe out through the mouth while making a 'huu' sound, also to the count of five. Gradually increase your counting periods to ten, fifteen and so on; or
- With your right thumb against your right nostril, breathe in smoothly through the left nostril to a count of five. Close the left nostril and hold the breath for a count of ten, then release the right nostril and breathe out to a count of ten. Then repeat the sequence starting with the left thumb against the left nostril.

Meditation

Meditation tends to have an aura of mystery about it, but it is something most of us do at some point in the day without realising. Meditation simply involves concentrating the mind on the task in hand to the exclusion of all else. That can be achieved by listening to a piece of music, making pastry, planning a business strategy or cultivating a blank mind while sitting cross-legged on the floor.

Focused meditation can be a powerful tool to expand consciousness and achieve the sort of insights and inner contentment which can ultimately help to relieve the effects of stress and anxiety. Western researchers have found that experienced meditators can reduce their heart rate and blood pressure as well as increase certain brain activity while meditating. These effects can obviously be extremely beneficial to well-being and health. Meditation has also been used to help reduce addictive behaviour – to alcohol, nicotine or recreational drugs.

Numerous techniques have been advocated to aid meditation. Staring at a candle or *mandala* (complex pattern) and concentrating the mind solely on that is one classic technique that is easier said than done by those with busy lifestyles and hectic schedules. Others urge deep breathing techniques, as with the yoga exercises described above. Guided meditation using tapes describing walks through a garden or the sound of waves breaking on a shore are also helpful for some. Others use the repetition of a *mantra* or sound: *Om* is often suggested from the Sanskrit phrase *Om mali padma hun* or 'the jewel in the eye of the lotus'.

Meditation – as usually understood in the West – demands quiet rooms, stillness, and no interruptions. Meditators are recommended to sit comfortably – on a chair if preferred, not necessarily cross-legged on the floor – and focus on their chosen meditation tool be that an image or sound. Using meditation to combat stress does not demand the sort of discipline and perfect motionless contemplation of a Buddhist monk – stretching, yawning, scratching are all permissible if the sitting position becomes just a little too uncomfortable. The length of time taken to meditate can be just as flexible – five minutes twice a day can be just as beneficial as an hour of inconvenient exercise.

A rather simpler 'practice' is described by Tenzin Palmo – an Englishwoman who became a Buddhist nun and spent twelve years meditating in a cave high in the Himalayas (Mackenzie, 1998):

> You can meditate walking down the corridor . . . waiting for the computer to change, at the traffic lights, standing in a queue, going to the bathroom, combing your hair. Just be there in the present, without the mental commentary. Start by choosing one action during the day and decide to be entirely present for that one action. Drinking the tea in the morning. Shaving. Determine, for this action I will really be there. It's all habit. At the moment we've got the habit of being unaware. We have to develop the habit of being present.

Typical of this approach is a technique called the half smile. All one need do is lift the corners of the mouth slightly – in a half smile – and hold the expression for the space of three breaths.

Repeating this six times or more each day – while waiting in a queue or staring at a computer screen – helps to encourage the sort of concentration and focus on the present that Tenzin Palmo describes. And it's all a great deal easier in a busy life than sitting staring at candles or chanting *mantras*.

Diet

Food also affects our ability to cope with stress and the impact those stresses have on our well-being. When we're stressed – as discussed earlier – the body starts to produce the 'flight or fight' hormone adrenaline, gearing it for action. Action needs energy so this adrenaline rush causes stored glucose to be drawn from the tissues in case it is needed. In the negative stress response this sugar remains unused so is converted back into fat and – since the sugar reserves are then depleted – means that we crave more food to restock the glucose cupboard.

The result is often excessive intake of chocolates and sweet drinks – easily seen most evenings on commuter trains, as stressed office workers munch their way through assorted snacks on the way home.

Caffeine-rich drinks can be a problem, too. While caffeine has a role in stimulating a sluggish system and may be helpful, in controlled doses, in depression or temporary tiredness, too many stimulant drinks during the day can compound the stress problem. Extra cups of coffee or cola drinks very quickly push up the caffeine intake (Table 9) and can cause palpitations, tremors, and

Table 9: Caffeine content of popular drinks

1 cup coffee	80mg
1 cup instant coffee	60mg
1 can (12 oz) cola	up to70mg
1 cup tea	50mg
1 cup cocoa	up to 40mg

raised blood pressure – easily increasing any underlying feelings of anxiety or tension.

The quantities given in the table are for standard tea *cups* not mugs – and certainly not the enormous quantities sold in popular American-style coffee bars as a 'small' latte. Limit coffee intake to no more than four standard cups daily.

Herbal, caffeine-free, alternatives are readily available: rooibosch (a South African herb) is ideal for those who like the taste of traditional Indian tea, while carob or commercially roasted-grain drinks make suitable substitutes for cocoa and coffee. Among the more popular herbal offerings look for those containing hibiscus, linden, vervain or wood betony. Decaffeinated drinks may seem ideal, but the caffeine is often extracted with chemical solvents which can leave unpleasant residues, so check labels and choose products that have been decaffeinated using water-based extraction methods.

Regular meals – including breakfast – are also important. Those with rushed over-worked lifestyles frequently miss this important start to the day leading to more imbalances in blood sugar and resultant increases in stress levels. Finding time to eat something first thing in the morning – even if it is just a sandwich on the train or a bowl of cereal on arriving at the office – really is important. Better still – invest in a slow cooker and brew your oatmeal porridge overnight so that it is ready to eat before you leave for work.

Feeling good

It is generally accepted that happy people are less likely to suffer from routine illnesses and tend to live longer: one American study suggests that people who look on the bright side of life actually have stronger immune systems. Studies on life expectancy show that people living alone tend to die sooner than those in a settled relationship while research into absenteeism suggests – rather obviously – that those who dislike their jobs are more likely to take days off work through ill health.

Being content and satisfied with what we have does not imply a return to some hierarchical society where we each stoically accept the cards fate deals us. It means clearly and consciously identifying what is important to us as individuals, setting our own agenda to achieve whatever these parameters may be, and then – rather than constantly moving the goal posts to a new ambitious target – being quite satisfied with what we have.

For many people a certain amount of stress is stimulating and enjoyable – one only has to watch journalists on a successful press day or dealers on a trading floor during a bull market, to see people happily responding to stress. Some obviously cope better than others and if you are one of those people who finds sudden peaks in stress levels worrying and exhausting then it may be time for a change.

Finding that much-wanted 'feel-good factor' need not involve mind-enhancing remedies and complex therapies – just a more relaxed attitude, a little herbal support, and a shift in emphasis from the pursuit of pleasure to happiness now.

References and further reading

References

Abramson, J., *et al.* (2001). *Ach. Int. Med.*, 161(14), 1725–30.

Abramova, Z. I., Chernyi, Z. K., Natalenko, V. P., *et al.* (1972). *Lek Sredstva Dal'nego Vostoka*, 11, 106–8, quoted in S. Mills and K Bone (2000). *Principles and Practice of Phytotherapy*, Churchill Livingstone, London.

Anand, C. L. (1971). *Nature*, 223, 496.

Bartram, T. (1995). *Encyclopaedia of Herbal Medicine*, Grace Publishers, Christchurch.

Bensky, S., and Gamble, A. (1986). *Chinese Herbal Medicine*, Eastland Press, Seattle.

Bone, K. (1996). *Clinical Applications of Ayurvedic and Chinese Herbs*, Phytotherapy Press, Queensland.

Boughton, F. (1998). *Australian J. Med. Herbalism*, 10 (2), 51–60.

Bradley, P. (ed.) (1992). *British Herbal Compendium*, BHMA, Bournemouth.

Bradwein, J., Zhou, Y., Koszychi, D., and Shlik, J. (2000). 'Placebo-controlled study of the effects of *gotu kola (Centella asiatica)* on acoustic startle response in healthy subjects', *J. Clin. Psychopharm.*, 20(60), 680–4.

Brekhman, I. I., and Dardymov I. V. (1969). *Ann. Rev. Pharmacol.*, 9, 419–30.

Broughton, A. (1999). 'The Sunshine Herb', *Eur. J. Herb. Med.*, 4(3), 29–33.

Broughton, A., and Denham, A. (2000). '*Hypericum* and drug interactions', *Eur. J. Herb. Med.*, 5(2), 19–25.

Brown,R. P., Gerbag P. L., and Ramazanov, Z. (2002). '*Rhodiola rosea:* a phytomedicional overview', *Herbalgram*, 56, 40–52.

Buchbauer, G., Jirovet, L., Jäger, W., Dietrich, H., Plnk, C., and Karamat, E. (1991). 'Aromatherapy. Evidence of sedative effects in the essential oil of lavender after inhalation,' *Z. Naturforsch*, 46c, 1067–72.

Chang, H., and But, P. (1986). *Pharmacology and Applications of Chinese Materia Medica, Vol. 1*, World Scientific, Singapore.

Conway, P. (2001). *Tree Medicine*, Piatkus, London.

Cook, J. (1777). *A Voyage towards the South Pole and Round the World*, Strahan & Cadell, London; Beaglehole, J. C. (ed.) (1961). *The Journals of Captain Cook: II The Voyage of the Resolutions and Adventure 1772–1775*, The Hakluyt Society, Cambridge.

Cooper, W. C., and James, J. (1990). *International Conference on AIDS, June 20–23, 1990*, 6(2), 369.

Dorling, E., Kirchdorfer, A. M., and Ruckert, K. H. (1980). *Notabene Med.*, 10(5), 241–6.

Duda, R. B., Zhong, Y., Navas, V., Li, M. Z. C., Toy, B. R., and Alvarez, J. G. (1999). 'American ginseng and breast cancer therapeutic agents synergistically inhibit MCF–7 breast cancer cell growth.' *J. Surg. Oncol.*, 72, 230–9.

Eagles, J. M. (2001). *Lancet*, 358 (9299), 2100.

Emerit, I., Arutyunyan, R., Oganbesian, N., *et al.* (1995). *Free Radic. Biol. Med.*, 18(6), 985–991.

Ernst, E. (2000). *Lancet*, 354(9195), 2014–16.

Escher, M., Desmeules, J., Glostra, E., and Mentha, G. (2001). 'Hepatitis associated with kava, a herbal remedy for anxiety', *Br. Med. J.*, 322 (7294), 1097.

ESCOP (1996). *Melissae Folium, Fascicule 2*, ESCOP, Exeter.

ESCOP (1997). *Valerianae Radix, Fascicule 4*, ESCOP, Exeter.

Foster, S. (1999). 'Black Cohosh. a literature review', *Herbalgram*, No 45, pp.35–45.

Foster, S., and Chongxi, Y. (1992). *Herbal Emissaries*, Healing Arts Press, Rochester, Vermont.

Frawley, D. (1989). *Ayurvedic Healing*, Passage Press, Salt Lake City.

Frawley, D. and Lad, V. (1988). *The Yoga of Herbs*, Lotus Press, Santa Fe.

Fulder, S. (1980). *The Root of Being. ginseng and the pharmacology of harmony*, Hutchinson, London.

Furgiuele, A. R., Kinnard, W. J., Aceto, M. D., *et al.* (1965). *J. Pharm Sci.*, 54, 247–52.

Gleitz, J., Friese, J., Beile, A., Ameri, A., and Peters, T. (1996). 'Anticonvulsive action of kavain estimated from its properties on simulated synaptosomes and sodium channel receptor sites', *Eur. J. Pharmacol.*, 315, 89–97.

Gleitz, J., Beile, A., Wilkens, P., Amdri, A., and Peters, T. (1997). 'Antithrombotic action of the kava pyrone kavain prepared from *Piper methysticum* on human platelets', *Plant Med.*, 63, 27–30.

Gorman, J. M., and Sloan, R. P. (2000). *Am. Heart J.*, 140(4), S77–83.

Grieve, M. (1931). *A Modern Herbal*, Jonathan Cape, London.

Guerin, J.-C., and Reveillere, H.-P. (1984). *Ann. Pharm. Fr.*, B, 553–9.

Guo, S. K., *et al.* (1983). *Planta Medica*, 48, 63.

Hänsel, R. (1968). 'Characterisation and physiological activity of some kava constituents', *Pacific Science*, 22, 293–313.

Herbalgram (1993). 'Mental function and *gotu kola,* research review', *Herbalgram*, 28, 32.

Herbs for Health (1998). 'Sage, rosemary, balm and more – the latest research on Alzheimer's', *Herbs for Health*, Jan/Feb 1998, pp. 48–51.

Hiai, S., Yokoyama, H., Oura, H., *et al.* (1979). *Endocrinol. Jpn.*, 26(6), 661–5.

Hofferberth, B. (1994). *Human Psychopharmacol.*, 9, 215–22.

Holden, R. (1998). *Happiness Now!*, Hodder & Stoughton, London.

Holmes, T., *et al.* (1967). 'The social readjustment rating scale', *J. Psychosomatic Res.*, 11, 213–18.

Hong, B., *et al.* (2002). *J. Urology*, 168(5), 2070–3.

Johnson, D., Frauendorf, A., Stecker, K., *et al.* (1991). *Neurologie Psychiatrie*, 5, 632–42.

Joyeux, M., Lobstein, A., Anton, R. *et al.* (1995). *Planta Med.*, 61(2), 126–9.

Kaminski, P. (1998). *Flowers that Heal,* Newleaf, Dublin.

Keji, C. (1981). *Am. J. Chinese Med.*, 9, 193.

Kohnen, R., and Oswald, W.-D. (1988). 'The effects of valerian, propranolol and their combination on activation, performance and mood of healthy volunteers under social stress conditions'. *Pharmacopsychiatry*, 21, 447–8.

Kovats, E. (1987). 'Bulgarian Oil of Rose (*Rosa damascena* Mil)', *Journal of Chromatography*, 406, 185–222.

Krishnan, K. R. R. (2000). *Am. Heart. J.,* 140(4), S70–6.
Kuppurajan, K., *et al. (*1980). *J. Res. Ayu. Sid.*, 1, 247.
Lane, H. C., and Fauci, A. S. (1985). *Ann. Intern. Med.*, 103(5), 714–8.
Leatherwood, P.D., Chauffard, E., Heck., E., and Munoz-Box., R. (1982). *Pharmacol, Biochem. Behav.*, 17, 65.
Lebot, V., Merlin, M., and Lindstrom, L. (1997). *Kava – The Pacific Elixir*, Healing Arts Press, Rochester, Vermont.
Lehmann, E., Kinzler, E., Friedemann, J. (1996). *Phytomedicine*, 3(2), 113–19.
Li, D., *et al.* (1987). *Henan J. of TCM*, 1, 29; English abstract *Traditional Chinese Medicine Digest*, 2(3–4), 41 (1987).
Lindahl, O., and Lindwall, L. (1989). *Pharmacol. Biochem. Behav.*, 32, 1065.
Linde, K., Ramirez, G., Mulrow, C. D., *et al.* (1996). *Br. J. Med.*, 313(7052), 253–8.
Lindstrom, L. (1981). 'Speech and kava on Tanna' in *Vanuatu. Politics, economics and ritual in island Melanesia*, ed. M. Allen, Academic Press, Sydney.
Mackenzie, V. (1998). *Cave in the Snow*, Bloomsbury Publishing, London.
Madge, T. (2001). *White Mischief – a cultural history of cocaine*, Mainstream Publishing, Edinburgh.
Maier-Hauff, K. (1992). World Congress of Medicinal and Aromatic Plants for Human Welfare, Maastricht, July 19–25, 1992.
McCaleb, R, (1990). 'Motherwort for the heart', *Herbalgram*, 22, 15.
McIntyre, A. (1996). *The Complete Floral Healer*, Gaia Books, London.
MediHerb (1996). 'Long-term kava therapy for anxiety', *MediHerb Monitor*, No 16 reported in *Greenfiles*, 10(1),16.
Mills, S. Y., and Bone, K. (2000). *Principles and Practice of Phytotherapy*, Churchill Livingstone, Edinburgh.
Morazzoni, P., and Bombardelli, E. (1995). '*Valeriana officinalis:* traditional use and recent evaluation of activity', *Fitoterapia*, 66 (2),99–112.
Muir, F. (1997). *A Kentish Lad*, Bantam Press, London.
Murch, S. J., *et al.* (1997). 'Melatonin in feverfew and other plants,' *The Lancet* 350 (9091), 1598–9.
Nalini, K., *et al.* (1992). 'Effect of *Centella asiatica* fresh leaf aqueous

extract on learning and memory and biogenic amine turnover in albino rats', *Fitoterapia*, 63(3), 232–7.

Newall, C. A., Anderson, L. A., and Phillipson, J. D. (1996). *Herbal Medicine*, Royal Pharmaceutical Society, London.

O'Connor, C. M., *et al.* (2000). *Am. Heart J.*, 140(4), S63–9.

Ody, P. (1989). 'Discovering the magic of rose oil', *The Herbal Review*, 14(3), 10–13.

Pearce, I. (1983). *The Gate of Healing*, Neville Spearman, Jersey.

Peigen, X., and Keji, C. (1987). *Phytotherapy Research*, 1, 53–7.

Physicians Desk Reference (PDR) for Herbal Medicines (2000), Medical Economics, Montvale, NJ.

Pietroni, P. (1990). *The Greening of Medicine*, Gollancz, London.

Pitzalis, M. V. *et al.* (2001). *Am. Heart J.*, 141(5), 765–71.

Roberts, A., and Williams, J. M. (1992). *Br. J. Med. Psychol.*, 65(2), 197–9.

Ryall, R. (1996). *The Magic of Herbs*, Capall Bann Publishing, Swansea.

Satyavati, G. V. (1988). *Indian J. Med. Res.*, 87, 327.

Schlieffer, H. (1973). *Sacred Narcotic Plants of the New World Indians*, Hafner Press, New York.

Scholing, W. E., and Clausen, H. D. (1977). *Med. Klin.*, 72 (32–3), 1301–6.

Schulz V., Hübner, W D., and Ploch, M. (1997). 'Clinical trials with phytopsychopharmacological agents', *Phytomedicine*, 4(4), 379–87.

Scruton, R. (2002). 'Still Burning', *The Business/Financial Times*, 19 January 2002, p.40.

Shan, B. E. *et al.* (1999). *Int. J. Immunopharmacolory*, 21 (3), 149–59.

Singh, Y. N. (1983). 'Effects on kava on neuromuscular transmission and muscle contractility', *Journal of Ethnopharmacology*, 7, 267–76.

Solomon, P. R. *et al.* (2002). *J. Amer. Med. Ass.*, 288(7), 835–40.

Spasov, A. A., Wikman, G. K., Mandrikov, V. B., Mironova, I. A., and Neumoin, V. V. (2000). 'A double-blind placebo-controlled pilot study of the stimulating and adaptogenic effect of *Rhodiola rosea* SHR–5 extract on the fatigue of students caused by stress during an examination period with a repeated low-dose regimen', *Phytomedicine*, 7(2), 85–9.

Speroni, E., and Minghetti, A. (1981). 'Neuropharmalogical activiy of extracts of *Passiflora incarnata', Planta Medica*, 54, 488–91.

Subhan, Z., and Hindmarch, I. (1986) *Int. J. Clin. Pharmacol. Res.*, 4(2), 89–93.

van Straten, M. (1993). *The Good Sleep Guide*, Kyle Cathie, London.

van Straten, M. (1994). *Guarana,* C W Daniel, Saffron Walden.

Svoboda, K. P., and Deans, S. G. (1990). *Variability of rosemary and sage volatile oils obtained from plants of various geographical sources and antioxidative properties of solvent extracts*, 21st International Symposium on Essential Oils, Lahti, Finland.

Thies, P.W. (1968). *Tetrahedron Letters,* 24, 313.

Tisserand, R. (1977). *The Art of Aromatherapy*, C W Daniels, Saffron Walden.

Torssell, K., and Wahlberg, K. (1967). *Acta Chem. Scanda.*, 21, 53.

Vuksan, V., Sievenpiper, J. L., Koo, V. Y. Y., Francis, T., Beljan-Zdravkovic, U. (2000). 'Post-prandial glycemia in non-diabetic subjects and subjects with Type 2 diabetes mellitus', *Arch. Intern. Med.*, 160, 1009–13.

Venkatraghavan, S., *et al.* (1980). *J. Res. Ayu. Sid.*, 1, 370.

Vogel, V. J. (1960). *American Indian Medicine*, University of Oklahoma Press, Norman.

Volz, H. P., and Kieser, M. (1997). *Pharmacopsychiatry*, 30, 1–5.

Viola, H., Wasowski, C., Levi de Stein, M., *et al.* (1995). *Planta Med.*, 61, 213–15.

Weiss, R.F. (1988). *Herbal Medicine*, translated from the 6th edition of *Lehrbuch der Phytotherapie*, Beaconsfield Publishers, Beaconsfield.

Wheatley, D, (1999). *Curr. Med. Res. Opin.*, 15(1), 33–7.

Whistler, Arthur (1992). *Polynesian Herbal Medicine*, National Tropical Botanical Garden, Hawaii.

Wiley, L. B.(1885). *Veterinary and Human Toxicology*, 37, 364–5.

Willard, T. (1990). *Reishi Mushroom: herb of spiritual potency and medical wonder*, Sylvan Press, Issaquah, Washington.

Woelk, H., Kapoula, O., Lehr, S. *et al.* (1993). *Z. Allg. Med.*, 69(10), 271–7.

Wohlfart, R., Hänsel, R., and Schmidt, S. (1983). 'The sedative-hypnotic principle in hops. 4. Communication: Pharmacology of 2–methyl–3-buten–2-ol'. *Planta Medica*, 48, 120–3.

Yanchi, L. (1988). *The Essential Book of Traditional Chinese Medicine*, Volume 1: Theory, Columbia University Press, New York.

Yun, T. K., and Choi, S. Y. (1995). *Cancer Epidemiol. Biomarkers Prev.*, 4(4), 401–8.

Zhu, B., *et al.* (1987). *Chinese Journal Integrated. Traditional and Western Medicine*, 7, 591.

Herbals

Bartram, T. (1995). *Encyclopaedia of Herbal Medicine*, Grace Publishers, Christchurch.

Bown, D. (1995). *Encyclopaedia of Herbs and their Uses*, Dorling Kindersley, London.

Chancellor, P. M. (1971). *Handbook of the Bach Flower Remedies*, C. W. Daniels, Saffron Walden.

Chevallier, A. (1996). *The Encylopedia of Medicinal Plants*, Dorling Kindersley, London.

Davis, P. (1995). *Aromatherapy. An A-Z*, 2nd Edition, C. W. Daniels, Saffron Walden.

Hoffmann, D. (1986). *The Holistic Herbal Way to Successful Stress Control*, Thorsons, Wellingborough.

Mills, S. Y. (1991). *Out of the Earth*, Viking, London.

Ody, P. (2000). *The Complete Guide. Medicinal Herbal*, Dorling Kindersley, London.

Ody, P. (2001). *Essential Guide to Natural Home Remedies*, Kyle Cathie, London.

Teeguarden, R. (1985). *Chinese Tonic Herbs*, Japan Publications, New York.

Weiss, R. F. (1988). *Herbal Medicine*, Beaconsfield Publishers, Beaconsfield.

Wren, R. C. (1988). *Potter's New Cyclopaedia of Botanical Drugs and Preparations,* C W Daniels, Saffron Walden.

Exercise therapies

Chen, Y. K. (1979). *Tai-Chi Chuan*, Newcastle Publishing, California.

Chia, M. (1986). *Iron Shirt Chi Kung I*, Healing Tao Books, New York.

Connor, D. (1992). *Qigong*, Samuel Weiser, Maine.

Dong, Y. P. (1993). *Still as a Mountain, Powerful as Thinder*, Shambala, Boston.

Liao, W. (1990). *T'ai Chi Classics*, Shambala, Boston.
Takahashi, M., and Brown, S. (1986). *Qigong for Health*, Japan Publications, Tokyo.
Yang, J.-M. (1988). *The Eight Pieces of Brocade*, Yang's Martial Arts Asociation, Jamaica Plain, MA.
Zhang, M., and Sun, X. (1985). *Chinese Qigong Therapy*, Shandong Science and technology Press, Jinan.

APPENDIX 1

Making herbal remedies

Infusions and decoctions

An infusion is simply a tea made by steeping the herb in freshly boiled water for ten minutes, while a decoction is a tea made by simmering the herb for longer and is the method used for tougher plant materials such as stems or bark.

Traditionally, herbal infusions were made once a day using ½–1oz (or 15–30g) of dried herb to 1pt (or 500ml) of boiled water and allowing the mixture to infuse for ten minutes, before straining and drinking the mix in three equal doses spread through the day. A decoction is generally made with ½–1oz (15–30g) of dried herb to 1½pt (750ml) of water reduced after about twenty minutes' simmering to 1pt (500ml). If using fresh herbs then you need three times as much because of the water content in the leaves.

A tisane cup (which has an inner ceramic pot with a strainer at the bottom) is ideal to use for making single doses of infusion; all herbal teas can be sweetened with a little honey if required.

Tinctures

A tincture is an alcoholic extraction of the active constituents of a herb made by soaking the dried or fresh plant material in a mixture of alcohol and water for two weeks and then straining the mix through a wine press or jelly bag.

Although any alcohol can be used to make tinctures, not all are safe to drink so great care needs to be taken with home production. Commercially produced tinctures are usually made from 95 per cent ethyl alcohol diluted to the required strength with water. Methyl alcohol is extremely poisonous and must never be taken internally, and although some recommend isopropyl alcohol (rubbing alcohol) for tincture making this is also very toxic and should be avoided. A more complex alcohol is glycerol or glycerine (propan–1,2,3–triol, available from chemists) which can be used and has the benefit of being very low cost, but the resulting tinctures are slightly slimy to the taste.

In many European countries the supply of high-grade alcohol is strictly controlled by state customs and excise departments, which can make home-made tincture production more complicated. A few are more flexible: in France, for example, it is possible to buy high strength, inexpensive, ethyl alcohol mixtures (around 45per cent or more) which are sold in supermarkets for bottling fruit, but in Britain and elsewhere the easiest way to obtain suitable alcohol for tincture making is to buy a basic quality vodka.

A 25 per cent alcohol/water mix is generally adequate for extraction of most herbs. This needs 25cl of alcohol and 75cl of water per litre. Vodka is usually 37.5 per cent alcohol (37.5cl of alcohol and 62.5cl of water per litre). To make this into a 25 per cent mix, you simply need to add an additional 500 ml of water to a 1 litre bottle of vodka.

Standard tinctures are usually made in the weight:volume proportion 1:5 (i.e. 1kg of herb to 5 litres of alcohol/water mixture). For home use mixing 100g of herb with ½ litre of the diluted vodka mixture is usually a sufficient quantity to make at any one time.

To make a tincture, simply put the required quantity of herb into a large jar, cover with the vodka/water mixture and store in a cool place for two weeks shaking the jar occasionally. Strain the mixture through a wine press or jelly bag and then store the tincture in clean, dark glass bottles. Tinctures will generally last for two years or more without deterioration.

APPENDIX 2

Glossary

adaptogenic – a herb that helps the body to adapt to strains and stresses by stimulating our own defence mechanisms; adaptogenics work with, rather than against, natural function.

alkaloid – active plant constituent containing nitrogen, which usually has a significant effect on bodily function.

analgesic – relieves pain.

anaesthetic – causes local or general loss of sensation.

anaphrodisiac – reduces sexual desire and excitement.

anodyne – allays pain.

anthroposophic – philosophy developed by Rudolf Steiner in the 1930s which teaches that health is related to internal vital force and energy.

antibiotic – destroys or inhibits the growth of micro-organisms.

anti-bacterial – destroys or inhibits the growth of bacteria

anti-fungal – destroys or inhibits the growth of fungi.

anti-inflammatory – reduces inflammation.

anti-microbial – destroys or inhibits the growth of micro-organisms.

anti-oxidant – prevents or slows the natural deterioration of cells that occurs as they age due to oxidation.

antiseptic – controls or prevents infection.

anti-spasmodic – reduces muscle spasm and tension.

aphrodisiac – promotes sexual excitement.

astringent – used to describe a herb which will precipitate proteins from the surface of cells or membranes thus producing a protective coating.

axil – in botany, the upper hollow where a lea or bract attaches to a stem.

bitter – stimulates secretion of digestive juices.

blood clotting – the process by which the proteins in blood are changed from a liquid to a solid by an enzyme, in order to check bleeding.

carminative – relieves flatulence, digestive colic and gastric discomfort.

catecholamines – group of physiologically important substances including **adrenaline**, **noradrenaline** and dopamine involved in the functioning of the nervous system.

cerebral circulation – blood supply to the brain.

choleric – one of the Galenic temperaments associated with yellow bile, heat and dryness.

circulatory stimulant – increases blood flow.

citronellal – a volatile oil with a lemon aroma found in a number of herbs and used for flavourings and insect repellents.

citronellol – a volatile oil with a rose-like aroma found in rose geranium and other species.

cleansing herb – a herb that improves the excretion of waste products from the body.

cooling – used to describe herbs that are often bitter or relaxing and will help to reduce internal heat and hyperactivity.

coumarin – active plant constituent which affects blood clotting.

depressant – reduces nervous or functional activity.

diaphoretic – increases sweating.

diuretic – encourages urine flow.

dosha – in Ayurvedic medicine one of the three essential substances which must be kept in balance to maintain health. Comparable to the 'humours' of Galenic medicine. See also **pitta**, **kapha**, and **vata**.

double blind study – A methodology for clinical trials where neither the patients nor those monitoring the results are aware of which medication, if any, is being administered.

eclectic – a herbal movement developed in North America in the nineteenth century.

essential fatty acids – a group of compounds of significant nutritional importance; lack of them is believed to contributary cause of arthritis, skin diseases, menstrual and menopausal problems and heart disease.

essential oil – volatile chemicals extracted from plants by such techniques as steam distillation; highly active and aromatic.

flavonoids – active plant constituents which improve the circulation and may have diuretic, anti-inflammatory and anti-spasmodic effects.

Galenic traditional Western medicine practised throughout Europe until the eighteenthth century and largely based on ancient Greek principles dating back to Hippocrates. The theory took its name from Galen, a Roman physician, and regards human health and temperament as controlled by four bodily humours: phlegm, yellow bile, black bile and blood giving rise to the temperaments: **phlegmatic**, **choleric**, **melancholic**, and **sanguine** (q.v.).

glucagon – a hormone released by the alpha cells in the islets of Langerhans in the pancreas which raises the blood sugar by stimulating the breakdown of glycogen in the liver to glucose.

hallucinogen – a substance which may cause hallucinatins.

hormone – a chemical substance produced in the body which can effect the way tissues behave. Hormones can control sexual function as well as emotional and physical activity.

humours – substances associated with bodily states or temperaments in both Galenic and Ayurvedic medicine. The Galenic humours were blood, yellow bile, black bile and phlegm. Ayurvedic humours are **vata**, **pitta**, and **kapha** (q.v.).

hypnotic – a substance that produces sleep by depressing brain function (also known as a sopoific)

kapha – phlegm, an Ayurvedic humour associated with earth and water elements.

Kirlian photography – a technique for capturing an image of the essential aura or energy field surrounding all living things. Developed by Semyon Kirlian in the 1960s.

melancholic – one of the Galenic temperaments associated with black bile, cold and dryness.

narcotic – a substance that induces stupor and insensibility and numbs pain,

nervine – herb that affects the nervous system and which may be stimulating or sedating.

neuroleptic – a substance capable of influencing psychotic symptoms, delusions and hallucinations.

neurotransmitter – a chemical substance released from nerve endings to transmit impulses across synapses to other nerves and across the minute gap between the nerves and the muscles or glands they supply. Major neurotransmitters include acetylcholine, **noradrenaline**, dopamine, serotonin, and gamma-aminobutyric acid.

noradrenaline – hormone related to adrenaline and with similar actions.
peripheral circulation – blood supply to the limbs, skin and muscles (including heart muscles).
phlegm – catarrhal-like secretion or sputum. In both Galenic and oriental medicine, phlegm is a more complex entity related in internal balance and sometimes associated with spleen deficiency.
phlegmatic – one of the Galenic temperaments associated with phlegm, cold and dampness.
photosensitivity – sensitive to light.
physiomedicalism – system of medicine developed in nineteenth century North America which focused on disease as a result of cold conditions.
pitta – bile, an Ayurvedic humour associated with the fire element.
polysaccharides – complex sugar molecules.
Qi (ch'i) – the body's vital energy as defined in Chinese medicine.
relaxant – relaxes tense and overactive nerves and tissues.
sanguine – one of the Galenic temperaments associated with blood, heat and dampness. It was regarded in the Middle Ages as the ideal temperament.
saponins – active plant constituents similar to soap and producing a lather with water. They can irritate the mucous membranes of the digestive tract which, by reflex, has an expectorant action. Some saponins are chemically similar to steroidal hormones.
sattva – in Ayurvedic medicine one of the three basic qualities of health (*gunas*) which can be translated as cognition or clarity; the other *gunas* are *rajas* – action and *tamas* – desire or substance.
sedative – reduces anxiety and tension.
simple – a herb used as a remedy on its own.
soporific – induces drowsiness and sleep.
stimulant – increases activity.
styptic – stops external bleeding.
thymoleptic – mood enhancing, anti-depressant.
thyroid – gland in the neck which controls metabolism and growth; it requires iodine for normal function.
tincture – liquid herbal extract made by soaking plant material in a mixture of alcohol and water.
tisane – an infusion.
tonic – restoring, nourishing and supporting for the entire body.

tonify – a tonic action: strengthening and restoring for the system.
topical – local administration of a herbal remedy.
vata – wind, an Ayurvedic humour associated with air and aether elements.
warming – a remedy which increases body temperature and encourages digestive function and circulation. Warming herbs are often spicy and pungent to taste.

APPENDIX 3

Suppliers and contact addresses

Associations and professional bodies

UK

British Herbal Medicine Association, Sun House, Church Street, Stroud, Gloucestershire GL5 1JL.

The General Council and Register of Consultant Herbalists. Marlborough House, Swanpool, Falmouth, Cornwall TR11 4HW.

The Herb Society, Sulgrave Manor, Sulgrave, Banbury, Oxon OX17 2SD.

National Institute of Medical Herbalists, 56 Longbrook Street, Exeter, Devon EX4 6AH.

The Natural Medicines Group, PO Box 5, Ilkeston, Derbyshire DE7 8LX.

USA

American Botanical Council, PO Box 210660, Austin, TX 78720.

American Herbal Products Association, PO Box 2410, PO Box 210660, Austin, TX 78720.

The American Herbalists' Guild, PO Box 1683, Soquel, CA 95073.

Northeast Herb Association, PO Box 266, Milton, NY 12547.

The Herb Research Federation, 1007 Pearl Street, Suite 500, Boulder CO 808302.

Australia

National Herbalists Association of Australia, Suite 14, 247–249 Kingsgrove Road, Kingsgrove, NSW 2208.

School of Herbal Medicine/Phytotherapy, PO Box 5310, Toowoomba, Queensland 4350.

Southern Cross Herbal School, PO Box 734, Gosford, NSW 2250.

Southern School of Natural Therapies, 43 Victoria Street, Fitzroy, Victoria 3065.

Victorian Herbalists Association, 24 Russell Street, Northcote, Victoria 3070.

Canada

Ontario Herbalists Association, 7 Alpine Avenue, Toronto, ONT M6P 3R6.

Herb suppliers

UK

G Baldwin & Co, 171–174 Walworth Road, London SE17 1RW.

East West Herbs Ltd, Langston Priory Mews, Kingham, Oxon OX7 6UW.

Hambledon Herbs, Court Farm, Milverton, Somerset TA4 1NF.

Jekka's Herbs, Rose Cottage, Shellards Lane, Alveston, Bristol BS35 3SY.

Neal's Yard Remedies, 26–34 Ingate Place, London SW8 3NS.

Cheshire Herbs, Fourfields, Forest Road, Little Budworth, Tarporeley, Cheshire CW6 9ES.

Chiltern Seeds, Bortree Stile, Ulverston, Cumbria LA12 7PB.

Iden Croft Herbs, Frittenden Road, Staplehurst, Kent TN12 0DN.

National Herb Centre, Banbury Road, Warmington, Nr Banbury, Oxon OX17 1DF.

Poyntzfield Herb Nursery, Black Isle, By Dingwall. Ross & Cromarty IV7 8LX.

USA

Bay Laurel Farm, West Garzas Road, Camel Valley, CA 93924.

Frontier, Box 299, Norway, Iowa 52318.

May Way Trading Chinese Herb Company, 1338 Cypress Street, Oakland, CA 94607.

Herbs Products Co, 11012 Magnolia Blvd., North Hollywood, CA 91601.
Kiehls Pharmacy, 109 Third Avenue, New York, NY10009.
Sage Mountain Herbs, PO Box 420, East Barre, VT 05649.

Australia

Australian Botanical Products Pty Ltd, 39 Melverton Drive, Hallam, Victoria 3803.
Blackmores Ltd, 23 Roseberry Street, Balgowlah, NSW 2093.
Greenridge Botanicals, PO Box 1197, Toowoomba Queensland 4350.
Essential Therapeutics, 6 Stuart Road, Lilydale, Victoria 3140.
Herbs of Gold Pty Ltd, 120 Milwood Avenue, Chatswood, NWS 2067.
Medi-Herb Pty Ltd, PO Box 713, Warwick, Queensland, 4370.
Southern Light Herbs, PO Box 227. Maldon, Victoria 3463.

APPENDIX 4

Plant names

This list provides a cross-reference of all relevant botanical and common herb names.

Achillea millefolium	Yarrow
Agaric	*Polyporus officinalis*
Agrimony	*Agrimonia eupatoria*
Alium sativa	Garlic
Aloe vera	*Aloe* spp.
Aspalathus linearis	Rooibosch
Amanita muscaria	Fly agaric
American ginseng	*Panax quinquefolius*
American valerian	*Centranthus ruber*
Angelica polyphorma var. *sinensis*	*Dang Gui*
Armoracia rusticana	Horseradish
Artemisia vulgaris	Mugwort
Ashwaghanda	*Withania somniferum*
Asparagus racemosus	*Shatavari*
Astragalus membranaceus	*Huang Qi*
Atropa belladonna	Deadly nightshade
Avena sativa	Oats
Balmony	*Chelone glabra*
Basil	*Ocimum* spp.
Bay	*Laurus nobilis*
Benzoin	*Styrax benzoin*
Black cohosh	*Cimicifuga racemosus*
Black hellebore	*Helleborus niger*
Borage	*Borago officinalis*

Calendula officinalis	Pot marigold
Californian poppy	*Eschscholzia californica*
Camellia sinensis	Tea
Cananga odorata	Ylang ylang
Cannabis sativa	Indian hemp
Cardamom	*Elettaria cardamomum*
Caterpillar fungus	*Cordyceps sinensis*
Catha edulis	Khat
Centella asiatica	Gotu *kola*
Centranthus ruber	American valerian
Chamaemelum nobile	Roman chamomile
Chamomile	*Matricaria recutita*
Chelone glabra	Balmony
Chocolate	*Theobroma cacao*
Cimicifuga racemosus	Black cohosh
Citrus bergamia	Neroli
Clary sage	*Salvia sclarea*
Claviceps purpurea	Ergot of rye
Cnicus benedictus	Holy thistle
Coca	*Erythoxylum coca*
Codonopsis pilosula	Dang Shen
Coffee	*Coffea arabica*
Cola nitida	Kola
Commiphora mukul	Guggul
Convallaria majalis	Lily of the valley
Cordyceps sinensis	Caterpillar fungus
Cowslip	*Primula veris*
Cramp bark	*Viburnum opulus*
Crataegus laevigata	Hawthorn
Crocus sativus	Saffron
Curcuma longa	Turmeric
Cyprepedium pubescens	Lady's slipper
Damiana	*Turnera diffusa* var. *aphrodisiaca*
Dan Shen	*Salvia miltiorrhiza*
Dang Shen	*Codonopsis pilosula*
Dandelion	*Taraxacum officinale*
Dang Gui	*Angelica polyphorma* var. *sinensis*
Datura stramonium	Jimson weed
Deadly nightshade	*Atropa belladonna*

Dioscorea villos	Wild yam
Elecampane	*Inula helenium*
Elettaria cardamomum	Cardamom
Eleutherococcus senticosus	Siberian ginseng
Ephedra sinica	*Ma Huang*
Ergot of rye	*Claviceps purpurea*
Erythoxylum coca	Coca
Eschscholzia californica	Californian poppy
Euphrasia officinalis	Eyebright
Evening primrose	*Oenothera biennis*
Eyebright	*Euphrasia officinalis*
Feverfew	*Tanacetum parthenium*
Fly agaric	*Amanita muscaria*
Ganoderma lucidem	*Reishi* mushroom
Garlic	*Alium sativa*
Ginger	*Zingiber officinale*
Ginkgo	*Ginkgo biloba*
Glycyrrhza glabra	Liquorice
Golden root	*Rhodiola rosea*
Gotu kola	*Centella asiatica*
Guarana	*Paullinia cupana*
Guggul	*Commiphora mukul*
Hawthorn	*Craetegus laevigata*
Helleborus niger	Black hellebore
Henbane	*Hyoscyamus niger*
Hibiscus	*Hibiscus sabdariffa*
Holy thistle	*Cnicus benedictus*
Honeysuckle	*Lonicera japonica*
Hops	*Humulus lupulus*
Horseradish	*Armoracia rusticana*
Huang Qi	*Astragalus membranaceus*
Humulus lupulus	Hops
Hyoscyamus niger	Henbane
Hypericum perforatum	St John's wort
Ilex paraguarensis	Yerba maté
Indian hemp	*Cannabis sativa*
Indian snakeroot	*Rauwolfia serpentina*
Inula helenium	Elecampane
Jamaican dogwood	*Piscidia piscipula*

Jasmine	*Jasminium grandiflorum*
Jimson weed	*Datura stramonium*
Jatamansi	*Nardostachys grandiflora*
Jati	*Jasminium grandiflorum*
Kava	*Piper methysticum*
Khat	*Catha edulis*
Kola nuts	*Cola nitida*
Korean ginseng	*Panax ginseng*
Lactuca virosa	Wild lettuce
Lady's slipper	*Cyprepedium pubescens*
Laurus nobilis	Bay
Lavender	*Lavandula angustifolia*
Lemon balm	*Melissa officinalis*
Leonurus cardiaca	Motherwort
Lily of the valley	*Convallaria majalis*
Linden	*Tilia cordata*
Ling Zhi	*Ganoderma ludicem*
Liquorice	*Glychrrhiza glabra*
Lonicera japonica	Honeysuckle
Lophophora williamsii	Peyote
Lotus	*Nelumbo nucifera*
Magic mushrooms	*Psilocybe* spp.
Ma Huang	*Ephedra sinica*
Marjoram	*Origanum majorana*
Matricaria recutita	German chamomile
Melissa officinalis	Lemon balm
Motherwort	*Leonurus cardiaca*
Mugwort	*Artemisia vulgaris*
Mullein	*Verbascum thapsus*
Myristica fragrans	Nutmeg
Nardostachys grandiflora	*Jatamansi*
Nelumbo nucifera	Lotus
Neroli	*Citrus bergamia*
Nicotiana tabacum	Tobacco
Nutmeg	*Myristica fragrans*
Oats	*Avena sativa*
Ocimum spp.	Basil
Oenothera biennis	Evening primrose
Opium poppy	*Papaver somniferum*

Origanum majorana	Marjoram
Panax ginseng	Korean ginseng
Panax quinquefolius	American ginseng
Papaver somniferum	Opium poppy
Pasque flower	*Pulsatilla vulgaris*
Passion flower	*Passiflora incarnata*
Paullinia cupana	Guarana
Peyote	*Lophophora williamsii*
Piper methysticum	Kava
Piscidia piscipula	Jamaican dogwood
Pot marigold	*Calendula officinalis*
Polyporus officinalis	Agaric
Psilocybe spp.	Magic mushrooms
Primula veris	Cowslip
Prunella vulgaris	Self-heal
Pulsatilla vulgaris	Pasque flower
Raspberry	*Rubus idaeus*
Rauwolfia serpentina	Indian snakeroot
Reishi mushroom	*Ganoderma lucidem*
Rhodiola rosea	Golden root
Rhubarb	*Rheum palmatum*
Roman chamomile	*Chamaemelum nobile*
Rooibosch	*Aspalathus linearis*
Rose	*Rosa* spp
Rosemary	*Rosmarinus officinalis*
Rubus idaeus	Raspberry
Saffron	*Crocus sativus*
Sage	*Salvia officinalis*
Salvia miltiorrhiza	*Dan Shen*
Salvia sclarea	Clary sage
St John's wort	*Hypericum perforatum*
Saffron	*Crocus sativus*
Sandalwood	*Santalum album*
Saw palmetto	*Serenoa repens*
Scutellaria lateriflora	Skullcap
Self-heal	*Prunella vulgaris*
Senna	*Senna alexandrina*
Serenoa repens	Saw palmetto
Shatavari	*Asparagus racemosus*

Siberian ginseng	*Eleutherococcus senticosus*
Skullcap	*Scutellaria lateriflora*
Stachys betonica	Wood betony
Stinging nettle	*Urtica dioica*
Styrax benzoin	Benzoin
Tanacetum parthenium	Feverfew
Taraxacum officinale	Dandelion
Tea	*Camellia sinensis*
Theobroma cacao	Chocolate
Thyme	*Thymus vulgaris*
Tilia cordata	Linden
Tobacco	*Nicotiana tabacum*
Turmeric	*Curcuma longa*
Turnera diffusa var. *aphrodisiaca*	Damiana
Urtica dioica	Stinging nettle
Valerian	*Valeriana officinalis*
Vervain	*Verbena officinalis*
Verbascum thapsus	Mullein
Viburnum opulus	Cramp bark
Wild lettuce	*Lactuca virosa*
Wild yam	*Dioscorea villosa*
Withania somniferum	Ashwaghanda
Wood betony	*Stachys betonica*
Yarrow	*Achillea millefolium*
Yerba maté	*Ilex paraguariensis*
Ylang ylang	*Cananga odorata*
Zingiber officinale	Ginger